Urban Emergency Medicine

Urban Emergency Medicine

Edited by

Mark Curato
Weill Cornell Medicine, New York, USA

Kaushal Shah
Weill Cornell Medicine, New York, USA

Christopher Reisig
Weill Cornell Medicine, New York, USA

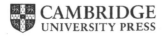

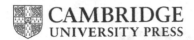

Shaftesbury Road, Cambridge CB2 8EA, United Kingdom

One Liberty Plaza, 20th Floor, New York, NY 10006, USA

477 Williamstown Road, Port Melbourne, VIC 3207, Australia

314–321, 3rd Floor, Plot 3, Splendor Forum, Jasola District Centre, New Delhi – 110025, India

103 Penang Road, #05–06/07, Visioncrest Commercial, Singapore 238467

Cambridge University Press is part of Cambridge University Press & Assessment, a department of the University of Cambridge.

We share the University's mission to contribute to society through the pursuit of education, learning and research at the highest international levels of excellence.

www.cambridge.org
Information on this title: www.cambridge.org/9781009181563

DOI: 10.1017/9781009181570

First published 2023

A catalogue record for this publication is available from the British Library.

A Cataloging-in-Publication data record for this book is available from the Library of Congress.

ISBN 978-1-009-18156-3 Paperback

Contents

Contributors

Doreen Agboh, MD
University of Chicago, Chicago, IL, USA

Surriya Ahmad, MD
NYU Grossman School of Medicine,
New York, NY, USA

Nicholas Avitabile, DO
Vagalos College of Physicians and
Surgeons, NewYork-Presbyterian/
Columbia University Medical Center,
New York, NY, USA

Jaskaran (Karan) Bains, MD, MBA
University of California, San Francisco,
CA, USA

Ahra Cho, MD
Icahn School of Medicine, New York,
NY, USA

Gregory R. Ciottone, MD, FACEP, FFSEM
Harvard Medical School, Beth Israel
Deaconess Medical Center, Boston,
MA, USA

Mark Curato, DO, FACEP
Weill Cornell Medical College, NewYork-
Presbyterian Hospital/Weill Cornell
Medical Center, New York, NY, USA

Stephen G. DeVries, MD, MPhil
Brigham and Women's Hospital and
Massachusetts General Hospital, Boston,
MA, USA

Elizabeth Dubey, MD, FACEP
Detroit Receiving Hospital, Wayne State
University School of Medicine, Detroit,
MI, USA

Devon Fiorino, MD
University of Chicago, Chicago, IL, USA

Scott A. Goldberg, MD, MPH, FACEP, FAEMS
Brigham and Women's Hospital, Boston,
MA, USA

Samita M. Heslin, MD, MBA, MPH, MA, MS
Renaissance School of Medicine at
Stony Brook University, Stony Brook
University Hospital, Stony Brook,
NY, USA

Trevor Marc Janus, MD
NYC Health + Hospitals-Lincoln Medical
Center, Bronx, NY, USA

Geoffrey W. Jara-Almonte, MD
NYC Health + Hospitals-Elmhurst
Hospital Center, Icahn School of Medicine,
New York, NY, USA

Michael P. Jones, MD
NYC Health + Hospitals-Jacobi/
Montefiore Medical Center, Albert
Einstein College of Medicine, Bronx,
NY, USA

Arvin K. Jundoria, MD, MHS
Johns Hopkins University School of
Medicine, Baltimore, MD, USA

Tammy Jupic, MD
Detroit Receiving Hospital, Wayne State
University School of Medicine, Detroit,
MI, USA

Marc Phillip Kanter, MD, FACEP
NYC Health + Hospitals-Lincoln Medical
Center, Bronx, NY, USA

Hemal Kanzaria MD, MSc
University of California, San Francisco,
CA, USA

Inkyu Kim, MD
Mass General Brigham, Boston, MA, USA

Dana Lauture, MD MS
Weill Cornell Medical College, NewYork-Presbyterian Hospital/Weill Cornell Medical Center, New York, NY, USA

David A. Leon, MD
Johns Hopkins University School of Medicine, Baltimore, MD, USA

Nisha Narayanan, MD
Weill Cornell Medical College, NewYork-Presbyterian Hospital/Weill Cornell Medical Center, New York, NY, USA

Alejandro A. Palma, MD, FACEP
Pritzker School of Medicine, University of Chicago, Chicago, IL, USA

Maria Raven MD, MPH, MSc
University of California, San Francisco, CA, USA

Christopher Reisig, MD, MA
Weill Cornell Medical College, NewYork-Presbyterian Hospital/Weill Cornell Medical Center, New York, NY, USA

Marimer Rivera-Nives, MD
NYC Health + Hospitals-Lincoln Medical Center, Bronx, NY, USA

Tony Rosen, MD, MPH
Weill Cornell Medical College, NewYork-Presbyterian Hospital/Weill Cornell Medical Center, New York, NY, USA

Kaushal Shah, MD, FACEP
Weill Cornell Medical College, NewYork-Presbyterian Hospital/Weill Cornell Medical Center, New York, NY, USA

Claudia Sofia Simich, MD
NYC Health + Hospitals-Jacobi/Montefiore Medical Center, Albert Einstein College of Medicine, Bronx, NY, USA

Laura Smylie, MD, FACEP
Detroit Receiving Hospital, Wayne State University School of Medicine, Detroit, MI, USA

Michael Stern, MD
Weill Cornell Medical College, NewYork-Presbyterian Hospital/Weill Cornell Medical Center, New York, NY, USA

Hanni Stoklosa, MD, MPH
Harvard Medical School, Brigham Health, Boston, MA, USA

Andrew Stolbach, MD, MPH
Johns Hopkins University School of Medicine, Baltimore, MD, USA

Reuben J. Strayer, MD
Maimonides Health, Brooklyn, NY, USA

Derrick Tin, MBBS
Harvard Medical School, Beth Israel Deaconess Medical Center, Boston, MA, USA

(Asa) Peter Viccellio, MD, FACEP
Renaissance School of Medicine at Stony Brook University, Stony Brook University Hospital, Stony Brook, NY, USA

Erena Weathers, MD
Icahn School of Medicine, New York, NY, USA

Preface

There is a mystique surrounding urban Emergency Medicine (EM). Medical students, physician assistants, EM residents, and attending emergency physicians all view "the big city" as a distinct practice environment – fast-paced, hard-edged, and unforgiving. The goal of *Urban Emergency Medicine* is to provide an expert-driven and clinically focused handbook for EM practitioners of all levels wishing to attain or improve upon their knowledge of how to work in an urban setting.

Urbanism involves large numbers of people concentrated in space, and those people inevitably are heterogeneous in terms of culture, language, economic status, and nearly every other variable that can differentiate persons and peoples. This amalgam comprising the human makeup of cities is fluid with mobility and transiency. The result is the concentration of certain social and physiological disease states, as well as the genesis and propagation of some uniquely urban challenges to health and healthcare delivery.

The mandate of EM specialist is to develop and maintain competence in the diagnosis and treatment of the acute phase of the entire gamut of illness and injury. The clichéd but undeniable truth is that the emergency physician must be ready for anything, and is therefore perpetually refreshing and renewing knowledge of rarely seen conditions, while honing and improving knowledge of common ones. Unarguably, this practice setting makes some things more common than others. *Urban Emergency Medicine* aims to unify the diseases, injuries, and practice barriers that are particular to the urban setting and to provide context, exposition, and tips for best practice from a group of authors who have spent their careers developing expertise in urban emergency medicine.

Chapter

1

Caring for the Homeless

Maria Raven, Hemal Kanzaria, and Jaskaran (Karan) Bains

Vignette 1

Forty-six-year-old unhoused man with a history of polysubstance use, including alcohol use disorder, presents with right-sided abdominal pain and tremors. The patient states that he has been drinking "almost a bottle" of vodka per day for the past 10 days, and his last drink was 7 hours ago. He states that he has felt similar pain multiple times in the past, and thinks it was also associated with heavy drinking. On initial evaluation, the patient is agitated and refuses to be examined, stating that he just wants to be left alone.

- What are the most appropriate next steps?
- What diagnostic testing should be ordered for this patient?
- How can you support this patient beyond acute clinical care while in the ED? Which Emergency Department (ED) team members should be involved in the care of this patient?

Vignette 2

Fifty-nine-year-old woman recently treated for pneumonia presents after a ground-level fall while walking with her son on the sidewalk. She was caught by her 32-year-old son but did strike her head on the grass. She states she has no medical history, takes no medications, and has never had any surgeries. She feels a bit weak but otherwise fine and is not interested in having laboratory tests drawn or staying in the hospital, as she states she has somewhere important to be. On exam, she is well-dressed and pleasant without acute findings, although she does have some conjunctival pallor from an unclear baseline. CT head and neck is negative.

- What is your differential diagnosis for this patient's presentation?
- What additional history would be useful to obtain from this patient?

Introduction

Despite its prevalence in society and particular salience in medicine, homelessness is not a well-understood term. Homelessness is driven by myriad structural forces, a reality that should be reflected in the language we use to describe our patients and others who lack housing. We will use the term "homeless" interchangeably with "person(s) experiencing homelessness" (PEH), "undomiciled," or "unhoused" throughout the text to emphasize that this patient population should not be stigmatized and defined solely by their housing status.[1]

1

Not only does homelessness encompass those who lack any fixed nighttime residence and those who reside in shelters or cars, but also multiple other groups not always considered homeless: those who are facing eviction within 14 days, who lack resources to maintain current housing for over 14 days with no subsequent housing plans, and who are fleeing domestic violence or other dangerous situations and lack resources for permanent housing.[2] Over 580,000 individuals experienced homelessness on a given night in 2020,[3] and cumulative estimates of those who experience homelessness during a calendar year approach 1% of the US population, or 3 million individuals.[4] There is enormous diversity within this population. Roughly one quarter of people experiencing homelessness are chronically homeless, defined as those who have a disability and have been homeless for 12 or more consecutive months or 4 or more separate occasions totaling at least 12 months over the past 3 years.[3,5] Two thirds of those experiencing chronic homelessness are unsheltered (compared to roughly half of the general homeless population) and are thus especially susceptible to negative health outcomes.[3] This group of unsheltered, chronically homeless individuals may be most likely to be identified as homeless upon presentation to the ED, despite comprising just 13% of the entire unhoused population.

Although homelessness affects all areas, nearly 60% of people experiencing homelessness are located in urban centers, with the vast majority living in one of the 50 largest US cities.[3] While many of the same structural factors affect homelessness regardless of location, there are meaningful distinctions between the rural and urban setting. Rural homelessness is more difficult to accurately estimate, with many unhoused individuals staying with family or friends as well as on wider expanses of land that facilitate remote living conditions.[6]

The geographical concentration of urban settings increases the visibility of homelessness to the entire population and can facilitate access to support services.[7] However, large numbers of unhoused individuals living in close proximity to each other often exceed the capacity of available services such as shelters. Urban homelessness is also exacerbated by stigma, higher construction costs, and complicated politics regarding construction of affordable housing.

Given the prevalence of homelessness in urban settings and the challenges faced by unhoused urban dwellers, it is essential that all urban emergency medicine clinicians be equipped to care for this population compassionately and effectively. Urban EDs experience a much higher proportion of visits from patients experiencing homelessness than national averages, which estimate that homeless patients make up 0.5% of total ED volume.[8] This is especially apparent in urban safety net hospitals, where over half of ED visits are by patients experiencing homelessness or other forms of housing instability in locations as disparate as Oakland and Atlanta.[9,10] Many homeless patients turn to these urban EDs when daily realities such as lack of a permanent address, identification, or insurance prove insurmountable barriers preventing them from accessing a healthcare system not tailored to their needs. By destigmatizing this patient population and learning best practices for their care, urban EM clinicians can improve outcomes for patients on each shift and mitigate the burn-out and helplessness that can arise from combatting the structural forces driving homelessness.

Structural Drivers of Urban Homelessness

The first step to providing effective care to people experiencing homelessness is addressing our own biases as clinicians by understanding the structural forces underpinning the homelessness crisis in the US. There is a large body of evidence supporting the claim that increasing scarcity of affordable housing is the main driver of urban homelessness. Analyses of Zillow data have indicated that rent affordability, or the share of income spent on rent, above 22% is associated with increased rates of homelessness. If rent affordability is above 32%, as in many major metropolitan areas across the nation such as New York City, Chicago, Los Angeles, San Francisco, Miami, Boston, and others, the rate of homelessness accelerates.[11,12] Increasing income inequality within urban centers can drive up housing prices and inflict disproportionately higher housing burdens on lower-income households, leading to increases in homelessness as well.[13]

This real estate competition from high-income households plays a central role in increasing urban demand for housing, while urban migration of people experiencing homelessness does not. Contrary to popular notions of mass migration of unhoused populations into cities, most people experiencing homelessness are doing so in the area they are originally from. In a study of homeless military veterans, only 15% of veterans receiving Veterans Administration (VA) homeless services migrated across large enough areas to switch VA service networks, and there were no net effects of migration on urban homelessness.[14] Similarly, a New York City (NYC) analysis revealed that 98.3% of families applying for NYC shelters in 2016 had a prior NYC address.[15] Other commonly cited causes of homelessness, such as mental illness or substance use disorders (SUDs), generally precipitate urban homelessness but do not directly cause it in the same systemic manner that housing inaccessibility does.[16]

While income inequality increases demand for housing, the lack of a supply side response is also highly culpable in the lack of affordable housing that drives urban homelessness. While building construction costs are higher in urban areas, local political resistance to constructing new housing units, particularly those labeled "affordable" housing, plays an even larger role in limiting housing supply. This phenomenon has given rise to the label NIMBY ("Not in My Backyard") to describe those who support the abstract concept of increased housing access as long as it does not affect their neighborhoods. This NIMBY activism has resulted in legal challenges to proposed housing developments across the country and across the aisle, with opposition from homeowners throughout the political spectrum.[17]

There are many forces underlying resistance to housing growth. Since the 1970s, when home appreciation outperformed stocks for the first time, homes increasingly became seen as investments. As a result, many homeowners began focusing all of their voting power on limiting housing growth to protect their home equity. Methods like single-family zoning laws, which prohibit lots from being used for any purpose other than single-family homes, were first used in urban settings to quash the possibility of low-income housing.[18] Homeowners were given veto power over new construction in their neighborhoods, an easy path to block new housing that persists today.

The common factor among these restrictive local land use policies is a foundation in racist ideology that continues to affect cities to this day. Single-family zoning laws were created with the intent of excluding people of color,[19] and racial covenants (many of which still exist in writing today despite being unenforceable) gave homeowners explicit legal basis to do so.[20] The practice of "redlining," which began in the 1930s, explicitly rated neighborhoods with black and immigrant populations as risky investments, regardless of actual mortgage default rates. The consequences of this racist policy, which precluded a generation of black Americans from obtaining home loans and other credit, continue to reverberate today in the form of compounding racial wealth inequality, particularly as home equity has become the primary source of generational wealth transfer in today's America.[21] Nearly 100 years after redlining was enacted, formerly redlined urban neighborhoods around the country are measurably hotter, more polluted, and have less green space than other areas.[22] Efforts to improve these conditions are often enacted only when gentrification is underway, further disadvantaging long-term residents who are largely people of color. The racial discrimination enshrined into the American housing system has been a major contributor to the overrepresentation of black and Indigenous individuals in the homeless population – in 2020, black Americans made up 39% of all people experiencing homelessness, but only 12% of the overall population.[3]

Characteristics of ED Visits by People Experiencing Homelessness

Patients experiencing homelessness have a high burden of disease. Although nearly one third of ED visits from this population are primarily for food, shelter, or safety,[23] their overall triage acuities and admission rates are not significantly different from patients with stable housing.[24] These patients are more likely to have acute psychiatric conditions or problems related to substance use that require emergency care. Furthermore, homelessness is independently associated with higher mortality even when controlling for poverty – the 21.7% 10-year mortality of sheltered homeless adults exceeded the 16.0% mortality of the lowest income quintile in one Canadian study.[25] These figures likely underestimate the difference in mortality between housed and unhoused populations, because unsheltered adults comprise 70% of deaths in the homeless population. The leading causes of death among people experiencing homelessness are acute intoxication and trauma, with homicide and suicide rates more than triple those in the general population.[26]

The US homeless population is aging, with a median age reaching 50 years in 2013 relative to 37 years in 1990. As patients experiencing homelessness who are 50 years of age or older have nearly twice the admission rates as their younger counterparts and are more likely to present with medical rather than psychiatric primary diagnoses, homelessness may become an even stronger risk factor for negative health outcomes in the future.[27]

Despite the high morbidity and mortality associated with homelessness, undomiciled patients experience longer ED wait times even when their presenting complaint is triaged as emergent.[28] Implicit bias, compassion fatigue, or even overt hostility toward patients experiencing homelessness may be contributing to this disparity. Many emergency clinicians also express concerns about the impact of patients experiencing homelessness on overall ED operations. While this patient population does have a higher proportion of psychiatric ED visits, which are more susceptible to ED boarding,[29] the impact of these patients is dwarfed by the overwhelming evidence that healthcare economics and wider systems issues drive boarding and other ED operational constraints.[30] Patients experiencing homelessness are generally aware of these disparities, which engender feelings of powerlessness, isolation, and stigmatization that damage the therapeutic relationship with clinicians from the outset.[31]

The negative impact of stereotypes on patients experiencing homelessness extends beyond the triage desk and into all aspects of patient care. Clinicians sometimes use biased pattern recognition, relying on characteristics such as hygiene, agitated behavior, and clothing to identify homeless patients rather than asking patients directly.[32] These heuristics are routinely employed by all levels of emergency clinicians, and are highly inaccurate given that five out of six undomiciled patients are sheltered or transiently homeless, as mentioned previously.

Simple practices such as routinely screening for housing status are high-impact when considering the increased burden of disease in patients experiencing homelessness, as well as the special considerations that must be incorporated into their care. For example, discharging a diabetic ketoacidosis patient with instructions to adhere to their medication regimen is unlikely to be effective if the patient does not have access to refrigeration for their insulin. Cephalexin, a common outpatient antibiotic for skin and soft tissue infections, may not be feasible for unsheltered patients to take four times daily as indicated, and alternate treatment may be more suitable. Emergency Department-based social services are also inaccessible to these patients unless they are properly identified. At a systems level, creating tailored solutions for specific homeless populations in any emergency department is unrealistic without obtaining an accurate scope of the issue. This failure to identify unhoused patients also limits the validity of data used in research on homelessness, hamstringing our ability to design effective policy.

Clinicians' hesitation to ask about housing status may stem from lack of training, personal discomfort, feelings of helplessness in addressing social determinants of health in the ED, or many other reasons.[33] Admittedly, there is no defined best practice for how to ask about housing, although experienced practitioners have introduced the topic with "Where are you staying these days?" and utilized follow-up questions as appropriate on a case-by-case basis.[34] Another important screening question for this population that is not always considered for stably housed patients is determining updated contact information, as many ED social services are ineffective without the ability to contact patients. Although over 90% of these patients have a cell phone, more than half have changed phones or phone numbers in the past 3 months.[35]

Using cognitive shortcuts also leads to deviations from the accepted standard of care. Homeless patients are less likely to be fully undressed for a physical exam, which can lead to missed injuries, sources of infection, or other pathology that is not readily apparent.[30,32] Given the many barriers to follow-up faced by unhoused patients, any acute or smoldering pathology may lead to significant morbidity and mortality if missed in the ED. Clinicians should have a low threshold for performing full physical exams on intoxicated patients in particular, as these patients may not be able to provide an accurate history. A team-based approach incorporating clinicians, nursing, social work, and other staff should be utilized if needed to facilitate such examinations.

Emergency Department-Based Interventions to Address Homelessness

In addition to providing high-quality clinical care, EDs can function as an access point for connecting the homeless population with support services that have been shown to measurably improve health outcomes. Emergency Department-based case management interventions, aimed at linking these patients with services such as shelter placement and psychosocial support, have proven effective at increasing housing and decreasing healthcare utilization in urban EDs, even by simply standardizing the deployment of existing social work resources for unhoused patients.[36] Case management has also demonstrated increases in health insurance, decreases in alcohol dependency, and increased primary care access in this population.[37,38] The use of peer care coordinators who have a history of homelessness has led to increased outpatient care utilization.[39] Yet despite a growing consensus on the cost-effectiveness of these programs,[40] budget limitations prevent their expansion in many EDs.

Interventions aimed at reducing substance use, such as overdose education and provision of reversal agents such as naloxone, have had mixed results. However, combining these initiatives with case management resources led to better outcomes, such as increased enrollment into substance use treatment.[38] The provision of reversal agents such as naloxone is a particularly promising area for ED intervention. However, low rates of unhoused patient follow-up preclude strong evidence on these "medications in hand" initiatives. Even small changes in clinician workflows to incorporate reversal agent provision proved significant barriers to initial implementation of this practice across multiple studies.[41]

While these interventions can be useful in combatting homelessness, the most crucial challenge for EDs to tackle remains access to housing. Although there is mixed evidence on the effects of housing programs on ED utilization, it is clear that such initiatives are highly effective in connecting homeless patients with housing.[38] In recent years, policymakers have begun to shift away from providing housing as an incentive for making lifestyle changes such as substance use reduction. "Housing first" programs, which operate under the well-founded assumption that housing is the major barrier to improved outcomes for homeless individuals, are becoming more common since the George W. Bush administration first incorporated them into federal policy.[42] In select states, Medicaid has begun covering services for formerly homeless residents in permanent supportive housing (PSH) over the past decade, lending further credence to the cost-effectiveness of Housing First.[43] Hospital systems have also invested in housing programs, aiming for the cost effectiveness, patient advocacy, and tax benefits of Housing First.[44]

Although much of the research on Housing First programs is limited due to small intervention size and varying study designs, there are promising signs that this approach is effective. A randomized controlled trial from California compared PSH with usual care for chronically homeless ED high-utilizers.[45] When combined with intensive case management services, PSH successfully placed 86% of patients in housing, with mean placement within 2.5 months and mean housing duration of over 2 years. Only 36% of homeless patients not provided with this service received housing. Moreover, the PSH group had lower utilization of shelters and psychiatric ED services. Permanent supportive housing was not associated with changes in overall ED or inpatient utilization.

The success of this wide array of ED interventions rests on matching services provided to the needs of the local homeless population and building trust with program participants. Even free housing programs can meet obstacles when the services provided diverge from participant needs, and organizations must have the agility to adjust. For example, a free COVID-19 isolation/quarantine hotel program in San Francisco, complete with a physician-supervised team of nurses and other healthcare workers that provided a wide range of support services to homeless patients, had a premature discontinuation rate of 19%.[46] Although the initial support team offered meals, opioid use disorder treatment, and symptom monitoring, it did not include multiple services needed by participants including mental health or telemedicine services and Americans with Disabilities (ADA)-equipped rooms. Meeting these needs may have improved retention. Mistrust of outreach workers and available services is also common among people experiencing homelessness,[47] underscoring the importance of building trust when promoting potentially beneficial policies such as those outlined in this section.

Assessing the Impact of Homelessness on ED Operations – De-Emphasizing ED Utilization

Many of the interventions discussed in the previous section have had tangible benefits for the unhoused population, from housing to reduced substance use. However, their impact on ED utilization is less clear. While ED utilization and costs are an important metric for resource-constrained hospital systems, ED costs are only a small component of overall healthcare spending.[48] Moreover, many ED-based interventions that help the homeless population have societal benefits that are not captured in ED data. Frequent ED users, many of whom are homeless, also use nonmedical public services such as shelters, mental health facilities, sober centers, and jail at a high rate. As a result, improved outcomes for this population may not be apparent unless utilization of all these sources is considered, a difficult task without integrated data.[49] Despite the absence of data-sharing infrastructure between these institutions, it is important to avoid falling into the tragedy of the commons by narrowing our view of this societal problem to the confines of the ED.

Health insurance provides an illustrative example. A plethora of research on Medicaid expansion under the Affordable Care Act demonstrates that patients with health insurance have better health outcomes.[50] Insurance expansion also addresses poverty and thereby homelessness. Twenty-two fewer evictions occur per year among every cohort of 1,000 new Medicaid enrollees relative to areas where Medicaid was not expanded.[51] Other factors contributing to homelessness, such as medical bills and loans, are also lower in insured populations. These changes are immensely valuable for patients, but insured status does not consistently decrease ED use by people experiencing homelessness. Analyses of both VA beneficiaries and Medicaid enrollees has shown that patients without stable housing are over six times as likely to be in the top 0.1% of ED utilizers or to name the ED as their usual source of care, respectively.[52,53] Despite being insured, these unhoused patients continue to use the ED frequently. Yet given the clear global benefits of increasing health insurance enrollment, ED utilization is not the primary outcome of interest in this setting.

Other interventions targeted toward the homeless population should be viewed through a similar comprehensive lens. Rather than focusing solely on measures of ED or healthcare utilization, ED leadership should recognize the positive externalities of combatting homelessness at a societal level and invest resources accordingly.[54]

Vignette 1 Conclusion

Patients like this man, who fit the "homeless" stereotype, can experience disparities in ED care right from triage, where they often wait longer than their housed counterparts of similar acuity. This patient's symptoms are consistent with alcohol withdrawal, and he may even be a frequent visitor to the ED. Regardless of the patient's history, the most appropriate next step is to assess whether the situation is safe to engage in a more extended discussion with the patient and communicate your concerns about his health. If the patient is too intoxicated or agitated to participate in his care, clinicians must use their clinical judgment to assess whether the need for a physical exam and/or testing are emergent enough to require the use of chemical or physical restraints. Restraints should be avoided if at all possible, and allowing patients to rest until they are more participatory is often the best course of action. In either case, the patient should be fully undressed and examined, just like any other ED patient. If the patient is able to provide a history, his housing status should be explicitly addressed.

Although alcohol withdrawal is high on this patient's differential diagnosis, his recurrent right-sided abdominal pain is also concerning for an acute intra-abdominal process, particularly when your abdominal exam reveals right upper quadrant tenderness to palpation. At this point, laboratory testing should be ordered, including a basic metabolic panel, complete blood count, liver function tests, and lipase. A right upper quadrant ultrasound would also be indicated given the location of the pain.

A bedside ultrasound shows multiple gallstones at the neck of the gallbladder, and labs are notable for a white blood cell count of 18, raising concern for the possibility of acute cholecystitis. This diagnosis may have been missed without a complete evaluation of the patient, beginning with a thorough physical exam.

While the patient is waiting to be evaluated by general surgery, you ask him if he is interested in resources for alcohol cessation. He states that he might be open to this. At this point, you should engage a multidisciplinary team to aid in the patient's care. If your institution has social workers and/or case managers, this would be an ideal time to involve them so that they can begin working on resources for the patient while he is in the hospital.

Vignette 2 Conclusion

In many cases, a patient with a low-impact traumatic head strike with negative CT imaging is reassuring. However, a more thorough social history is crucial in this patient. Although she does not fit the stereotypical appearance of an unhoused individual, on further questioning she states that she has been living in her car with her son for the past three weeks after they were evicted from their apartment. As a result, she and her son fall under the "homeless" category laid out by the US Department of Housing and Urban Development. She has not been eating her typical quantity of food during this time, which has contributed to her weakness, and she has not felt "normal" since she was treated for pneumonia three weeks ago.

These new findings are concerning and, in combination with her conjunctival pallor, they prompt basic lab testing with a basic metabolic panel and complete blood count. When the labs result, her hemoglobin is 3.7 but hemolyzed, and the patient is now reiterating that she feels fine and would like to leave.

At this point, the differential diagnosis for her anemia is wide and includes internal hemorrhage, gastrointestinal (GI) bleeding, severe iron deficiency anemia, B12 or folate deficiency, and hemolysis, among others. Given the presence of multiple life-threatening entities on this list, it is imperative to discuss your concerns with the patient and redraw a complete blood count along with labs to assess for hemolysis and iron studies.

The second hemoglobin value is the same as the first, and you decide to transfuse the patient and admit her to the hospital for further workup. On chart review a few days later, you see that the patient had a hemolytic anemia secondary to a prior atypical pneumonia, and is now doing well after multiple transfusions. Although she did not "look" homeless, her housing status placed her at high risk for increased morbidity, and your screening questions directly led to appropriate management for this patient.

Pro-Tips

- Although homelessness is a nationwide problem, it is particularly salient in the urban ED setting, where patients experiencing homelessness can make up over half of ED visits in some safety net hospitals.
- The most important factor driving homelessness is scarcity of affordable housing (rooted in a legacy of racism and discrimination), not mass migration, substance use, or other personal characteristics. Emergency Department clinicians should keep this in mind when treating unhoused patients in order to provide equitable care and avoid stigmatizing homelessness.
- Patients experiencing homelessness have a higher burden of disease than the general population, yet face barriers to care starting at ED triage. Emergency Department clinicians should be cognizant of the increased vulnerability of these patients when placed in the waiting room with high-acuity complaints.
- As a routine part of care for all patients, ED clinicians should ask about housing status instead of relying on pattern recognition to identify homeless patients, as the majority of patients in this category do not fit the stereotypes clinicians associate with homelessness.
- Emergency Department clinicians should ensure that these patients are undressed and obtain the full set of physical exam findings relevant to their presenting complaint. If the patient has altered mental status or is otherwise unable to provide sufficient history, clinicians should err on the side of a more thorough examination given the high medical risk and poor follow-up of this population.
- Emergency Department interventions such as case management services and housing programs can be immensely helpful for this population. These programs should be measured by not only their impact on ED utilization but also the more global health and wellness outcomes of patients.
- Tailoring interventions to address the specific needs of an ED's homeless patient population is a crucial prerequisite to successful ED-based interventions in this area.

References

1. Rich J. People Experience Homelessness, They Aren't Defined by It. 2017. www.usich.gov/news/people-experience-homelessness-they-arent-defined-by-it/ (accessed February 10, 2022).

2. Cornell Legal Information Institute. 42 US Code § 11302 – General definition of homeless individual. www.law.cornell.edu/uscode/text/42/11302.

3. The 2020 Annual Homeless Assessment Report (AHAR) to Congress. US Department of Housing and Urban Development. 2020. www.huduser.gov/portal/sites/default/files/pdf/2020-AHAR-Part-1.pdf (accessed February 9, 2022).

4. Strategic Action Plan on Homelessness. US Department of Health and Human Services. 2007. www.hhs.gov/programs/social-services/homelessness/research/strategic-action-plan-on-homelessness/index.html (accessed February 9, 2022).

5. 24 C.F.R. Parts 91 and 578; Final Rule: Homeless Emergency Assistance and Rapid Transition to Housing: Defining "Chronically Homeless." Federal Register 2015;80(233):75791–75806.

6. Meehan M. Unsheltered and Uncounted: Rural America's Hidden Homeless. NPR. 2019. www.npr.org/sections/health-shots/2019/07/04/736240349/in-rural-areas-

homeless-people-are-harder-to-find-and-
to-help (accessed February 10, 2022).

7. Tsai J, Link B, Rosenheck RA, Pietrzak RH.
    Homelessness among a nationally
    representative sample of US veterans:
    prevalence, service utilization, and
    correlates. *Social Psychiatry Psychiatr
    Epidemiol.* 2016;51:907–916.

8. Tadros A, Layman SM, Pantaleone
    Brewer M, Davis SM. A 5-year
    comparison of ED visits by homeless and
    nonhomeless patients. *Am J Emerg Med.*
    2016;34(5):805–808.

9. Fraimow-Wong L, Sun J, Imani P,
    Haro D, Alter HJ. Prevalence and
    temporal characteristics of housing
    needs in an urban emergency
    department. *West J Emerg Med.* 2021; 22
    (2):204–212.

10. Jackson TS, Moran T, Lin J, Sahi BA.
    Prevalence of homelessness and housing
    insecurity in an urban emergency
    department. *Ann Emerg Med.* 2017;70
    (4_suppl):S167.

11. Glynn C. Homelessness Rises Faster Where
    Rent Exceeds a Third of Income. Zillow.
    2018. www.zillow.com/research/homeless
    ness-rent-affordability-22247/ (accessed
    February 10, 2022).

12. O'Brien S, Schoen J. Here's the share of
    income that goes to rent in cities across the
    country. CNBC. 2019. www.cnbc.com/201
    9/03/07/heres-the-share-of-income-that-
    goes-to-rent-in-cities-across-the-us.html
    (accessed February 10, 2022).

13. Byrne T, Henwood BF, Orlando AW.
    A rising tide drowns unstable boats: how
    inequality creates homelessness. *Annals
    AAPSS.* 2021;693:28–45.

14. Metraux S. Migration by Veterans who
    Receive VA Homeless Services. US
    Department of Veterans Affairs. 2015. ww
    w.nchv.org/images/uploads/MigrationByV
    eteransReceivingHomelessServices_Oc
    t2015.pdf (accessed February 10, 2022).

15. Turning the Tide on Homelessness in
    New York City. NYC.gov. 2017. www1
    .nyc.gov/assets/dhs/downloads/pdf/turn
    ing-the-tide-on-homelessness.pdf
    (accessed February 10, 2022).

16. Resnikoff N. How the Atlantic's Big Piece
    on Meth and Homelessness Gets It Wrong.
    UCSF Benioff Homelessness and Housing
    Initiative. 2021. https://homelessness
    .ucsf.edu/blog/how-atlantics-big-piece-
    meth-and-homelessness-gets-it-wrong
    (accessed February 12, 2022).

17. Badger E. The Bipartisan Cry of "Not in My
    Backyard." *New York Times.* 2018. www
    .nytimes.com/2018/08/21/upshot/home-
    ownership-nimby-bipartisan.html
    (accessed February 11, 2022).

18. Dougherty C. *Golden Gates: The Housing
    Crisis and a Reckoning for the American
    Dream.* Penguin Books, 2021.

19. Resnikoff N. It's Hard to Have Faith in
    a State That Can't Even House Its People.
    New York Times. 2021. www.nytimes.com
    /2021/07/26/opinion/homelessness-
    california.html (accessed February 11,
    2022).

20. Thompson C. Racial Covenants, A Relic of
    the Past, Are Still on the Books Across the
    country. NPR. 2021. www.npr.org/2021/1
    1/17/1049052531/racial-covenants-
    housing-discrimination (accessed
    February 12, 2022).

21. Miller G. Newly Released Maps Show How
    Housing Discrimination Happened.
    National Geographic. 2016. www
    .nationalgeographic.com/history/article/h
    ousing-discrimination-redlining-maps
    (accessed February 11, 2022).

22. Plumer B, Popovich N. How Decades of
    Racist Housing Policy Left Neighborhoods
    Sweltering. *New York Times.* 2020. www
    .nytimes.com/interactive/2020/08/24/cli
    mate/racism-redlining-cities-global-
    warming.html (accessed February 12,
    2022).

23. Rodriguez R, Fortman J, Chee C, Ng V,
    Poon D. Food, shelter, and safety needs
    motivating homeless persons' visits to an
    urban emergency department. *Ann Emerg
    Med.* 2009;53(5):598–602.

24. Ku B, Scott KC, Kertesz SG, Pitts SR.
    Factors associated with use of urban
    emergency departments by the US
    Homeless Population. *Public Health Rep.*
    2010;125(3):398–405.

25. Hwang S, Wilkins R, Tjepkema M, O'Campo PJ, Dunn JR. Mortality among residents of shelters, rooming houses, and hotels in Canada: 11 year follow-up study. *BMJ*. 2009;339:b4036.

26. Cawley C, Kanzaria HK, Kushel M, Raven MC, Zevin B. Mortality among people experiencing homelessness in San Francisco 2016–2018. *J Gen Internal Med*. 2022;37:990–991. DOI 10.1007/s11606-021-06769-7.

27. Brown R, Steinman M. Characteristics of emergency department visits by older versus younger homeless adults in the United States. *Am J Public Health*. 2013;103 (6):1046–1051.

28. Ayala A, Tegtmeyer K, Atassi G, Powell E. The effect of homelessness on patient wait times in the emergency department. *J Emerg Med*. 2021;60(5):661–668.

29. Nolan J, Fee C, Cooper BA, Rankin SH, Blegen MA. Psychiatric boarding incidence, duration, and associated factors in United States emergency departments. *J Emerg Nursing*. 2015;41(1):57–64.

30. Kelen G, Wolfe R, D'Onofrio G, Mills AM, Diercks D, Stern SA, Wadman MC, Sokolove PE. Emergency department crowding: the canary in the health care system. *NEJM Catalyst*. 2021; DOI 10.1056/CAT.21.0217.

31. McCallum R, Medved MI, Hiebert-Murphy D, Distasio J, Sareen J, Chateau D. Fixed nodes of transience: narratives of homelessness and emergency department use. *Qual Health Res*. 2020;30(8):1183–1195.

32. Doran K, Vashi AA, Platis S, Curry LA, Rowe M, Gang M, Vaca FE. Navigating the boundaries of emergency department care: addressing the medical and social needs of patients who are homeless. *Am J Public Health*. 2013;103(S2):S355–360.

33. Raven M. Homelessness and the practice of emergency medicine: challenges, gaps in care, and moral obligations. *Ann Emerg Med*. 2019;74(5S):S33–37.

34. Salhi B, Doran K. Homelessness. In Alter H, Dalawari P, Doran KM, Raven MC (eds.). *Social Emergency Medicine*. Springer Nature, 2021.

35. Rhoades H, Wenzel S, Rice E, Winetrobe H, Henwood B. No digital divide? Technology use among homeless adults. *J Social Distress Homelessness*. 2017;26(1):73–77.

36. McCormack RP, Hoffman LF, Wall SP, Goldfrank LR. Resource-limited, collaborative pilot intervention for chronically homeless, alcohol-dependent frequent emergency department users. *Am J Public Health*. 2013;103(S2):S221–224.

37. Shumway M, Boccellari A, O'Brien K, Okin RL. Cost-effectiveness of clinical case management for ED frequent users: results of a randomized trial. *Am J Emerg Med*. 2008;26(2):155–164.

38. Formosa EA, Kishimoto V, Orchanian-Cheff A, Hayman K. Emergency department interventions for homelessness: a systematic review. *Canadian J Emerg Med*. 2021;23:111–122.

39. Nossel IR, Lee RJ, Isaacs A, Herman DB, Marcus SM, Essock SM. Use of peer staff in a critical time intervention for frequent users of a psychiatric emergency room. *Psychiatr Services*. 2016;67(5):479–481.

40. Kumar GS, Klein R. Effectiveness of case management strategies in reducing emergency department visits in frequent user patient populations: a systematic review. *J Emerg Med*. 2013;44(3):717–729.

41. Gunn AH, Smothers ZPW, Schramm-Sapyta N, Freiermuth CE, MacEachern M, Muzyk AJ. The emergency department as an opportunity for naloxone distribution. *West J Emerg Med*. 2018;19(6):1036–1042.

42. Resnikoff N. Housing First Is Not Housing Only. UCSF Benioff Homelessness and Housing Initiative. 2021. https://home lessness.ucsf.edu/blog/housing-first-not-housing-only (accessed February 13, 2022).

43. Cassidy A. Medicaid and permanent supportive housing. *Health Affairs*. 2016; DOI 10.1377/hpb20161014.734003.

44. Bartolone P. Hospitals invest in housing for homeless to reduce ER visits. *Healthcare Finance*. 2017. www .healthcarefinancenews.com/news/hos pitals-invest-housing-homeless-reduce-er- visits (accessed February 13, 2022).

45. Raven MC, Niedzwiecke MJ, Kushel M. A randomized trial of permanent supportive housing for chronically homeless persons with high use of publicly funded services. *Health Services Res.* 2020;55(S2):797–806.

46. Fuchs JD, Clay HC, Evans J, Graham-Squire D, Imbert E, Bloome J, Fann C, Skotnes T, Sears J, Pfeifer-Rosenblum R, Moughamian A, Eveland J, Reed A, Borne D, Lee M, Rosenthal M, Jain V, Bobba N, Kushel M, Kanzaria HK. Assessment of a hotel-based COVID-19 isolation and quarantine strategy for persons experiencing homelessness. *JAMA Netw Open*. 2021;4(3):e210490.

47. Kryda A, Compton M. Mistrust of outreach workers and lack of confidence in available services among individuals who are chronically street homeless. *Community Mental Health J.* 2009;45 (2):144–150.

48. Doran K, Boyer A, Raven M. Health care for people experiencing homelessness – what outcomes matter? *JAMA Netw Open*. 2021;4(3):e213837.

49. Kanzaria HK, Niedzwiecki M, Cawley CL, Chapman C, Sabbagh SH, Riggs E, Chen AH, Martinez MX, Raven MC. Frequent emergency department users: focusing solely on medical utilization misses the whole person. *Health Aff (Millwood)*. 2019;38(11):1866–1875.

50. Mazurenko O, Balio CP, Agarwal R, Carroll AE, Menachemi N. The effects of Medicaid expansion under the ACA: a systematic review. *Health Aff (Millwood)*. 2018;37(6):944–950.

51. Allen HL, Eliason E, Zewde N, Gross T. Can Medicaid expansion prevent housing evictions? *Health Affairs* 2019;38(9):1451–1457.

52. Doran K, Raven M, Rosenheck R. What drives frequent emergency department use in an integrated health system? National data from the Veterans Health Administration. *Ann Emerg Med*. 2013;62 (2):151–159.

53. Raven MC, Billings JC, Goldfrank KR, Manheimer ED, Gourevitch MN. Medicaid patients at high risk for frequent hospital admission: real-time identification and remediable risks. *J Urban Health*. 2009;86:230–241.

54. Kanzaria H, HoffmanJ. Hot-spotters aren't "the problem" . . . but they are emblematic of the failure of US healthcare. *J Gen Internal Med*. 2016;32(1):6–8.

Chapter 2

Disruptive and Dangerous Agitation

Reuben J. Strayer

Vignette

It's 4:30 a.m. on a Sunday morning, and the prehospital notification phone rings. Emergency Medical Services (EMS) will be arriving in 6 minutes with a man in his 30s. 911 was called to a dance club when a patron became agitated and violent. Presently, the patient is subdued by two basic life support (BLS) medics and four police officers, and the patient is in handcuffs, but still thrashing and incoherent. No vitals are obtainable, and BLS does not establish IV access or administer medications.

- How can this patient be safely approached and calmed? What is the role of physical restraints?
- What are the most important dangerous conditions to identify in the initial phase of care?

Introduction

Undifferentiated severe agitation is one of the clinical presentations in which emergency medicine clinicians are particularly expert. The patient suffering dangerous agitation of uncertain cause is squarely a prehospital and emergency department challenge – in fact a set of simultaneous challenges.

Dangerous agitation is seen infrequently in most centers and rarely outside of urban areas. Because cities focus the availability of illicit drugs of abuse, people with substance use disorders are prevalent in metropolitan areas. Untreated mental illness, the second major underlying factor driving dangerous agitation, is also more likely to occur in cities. Social disadvantage, especially homelessness and camps of people experiencing homelessness, concentrate the settlement of individuals with psychiatric disease and the distribution of street drugs, further promoting the development of behavioral disturbance and agitation. These three unfortunate features of city life – street drugs, mental illness, and homelessness – result in severe agitation as an urban disease.

The patient with undifferentiated, severe agitation is an immediate threat to himself and to clinicians, other personnel involved with their care, and anyone else in physical proximity, and this threat must be promptly and effectively managed by administering powerful drugs and often also simultaneously using dangerous physical restraint maneuvers. At the same time that control is being established and the risks of these drugs and maneuvers are being assessed and managed, the patient must be evaluated and treated for a range of threats to life that may be the cause of their agitation, or the result of their agitation and attempts by the public, law enforcement, or other clinicians to control it. All this occurs as clinicians are subjected to the risk of physical harm and verbal abuse from the patient they are treating, which poses an obstacle to providing effective care. The dangerously agitated patient must be simultaneously controlled, resuscitated, and risk stratified as they threaten the safety and mindset of the provider team.

Agitation may be stratified to three levels of severity, each indicating a different intensity of care.

(1) *Agitated but cooperative* patients respond to suggestion and may be managed with minimal or gentle pharmacology.

(2) *Disruptive without danger* patients require medications to treat their agitation but are not an immediate threat or threatened.

(3) *Dangerous agitation* is a medical emergency that requires immediate control to protect the patient and others, and to identify and treat associated dangerous conditions.

Agitated but Cooperative

The agitated but cooperative patient calms when engaged, is persistently verbally redirectable, and can participate in their own care. Common examples include a mildly demented older person, a mildly psychotic person with schizophrenia, or a mildly intoxicated teenager who should have been taken home but was brought to the emergency department (ED) instead. These patients can be reliably assessed by history and physical exam, and concern for an underlying dangerous condition is low.

These patients are usually easily managed by keeping them occupied, so the optimal strategy is to have someone (a relative, a volunteer, a med student) sit with them, engage and interact with them. Feeding these patients, reducing environmental stimulation, giving them access to video or audio media, and demonstrating reassurance and kindness may be enough to maintain a peaceful demeanor. Consider and treat reversible causes of mild agitation such as pain, full bladder, hunger, or thirst.

If pharmacologic treatment is required, the first choice is a medication the patient already takes or is known to be effective; otherwise, small doses of calming medications generally suffice. These medications should be offered by mouth or oral dissolving tablet, if possible. Second-generation antipsychotic agents are first-line in most cases; risperidone (0.25–2 mg PO) may be superior to the more anticholinergic olanzapine (2.5–10 mg PO), although both have demonstrated efficacy.[1] Ziprasidone may also be used (10–20 mg IM), although it is available only as a solution for IM injection that requires reconstitution, has a delayed effect compared to droperidol and olanzapine, is associated with more respiratory depression than alternatives, and may be teratogenic.[2] Aripiprazole has been demonstrated to be less effective than alternatives and quetiapine is disfavored for orthostatic hypotension.[3] Benzodiazepines can cause worsening delirium, especially in elderly patients, but are otherwise effective and safe when respiratory depression is not a concern. Oral lorazepam is typically dosed at 0.5–2 mg for mild agitation.

Disruptive Without Danger

In many urban emergency departments, the intoxicated, moderately agitated patient is a routine presentation. These patients are not easily redirected like the cooperative patients, but they are at least intermittently able to be engaged and, therefore, able to be reliably assessed. After this assessment, it is determined that drug intoxication (usually) is the diagnosis and that the patient is very unlikely to be harboring a dangerous condition. However, these patients are often loud and disruptive, and their moderate agitation requires active management. Although treatment of their agitation with medications is often required, verbal de-escalation should usually be attempted first, as described in Table 2.1.[4]

If verbal de-escalation fails, these patients require calming medications, as their agitation interferes with the care of other patients. The use of sedating medications to treat agitation is a trade-off between efficacy and safety, and because there is low concern for a dangerous condition in this group, the management priority tilts to safety. It is prudent to accept a delay to sedation and to accept the prospect of repeat medication administration, because (while frustrating) the disruption poses no danger, and thus avoiding medication harms is a central concern.

In this vein, the classic agitation cocktail, haloperidol 5 mg and lorazepam 2 mg, combined in the same syringe and injected intramuscularly, has the virtue of a wide margin of safety. "5 and 2" is very safe, and will be effective in most patients, eventually. However, sedation after 5 and 2 rarely occurs within 10 minutes, and often takes 15–20 minutes, because haloperidol is relatively slow-acting, and lorazepam is erratically absorbed intramuscularly.

Droperidol and midazolam, congeners in the butyrophenone and benzodiazepine class, are modestly more effective than haloperidol and lorazepam, but significantly faster, with a similar safety profile, and are therefore better choices in the management of moderate agitation in the ED.

The first-generation antipsychotic droperidol is more potent and more sedating than haloperidol, and has been used primarily for postoperative nausea and vomiting for decades. Droperidol has been repeatedly demonstrated to be safe and effective in the management of undifferentiated emergency agitation and is particularly well-suited to manage agitation associated with alcohol intoxication, as it is associated with less

Table 2.1 Verbal De-Escalation Techniques

De-Escalation Technique	Examples
Respect patient's autonomy	Utilize periods of intent listening Respect personal space
Introduce yourself and orient the patient	Emphasize to the patient that you are their medical provider to help care for them, and that they are in a hospital setting
Identify wants or needs	Offer comfort objects (warm blankets) Facilitate using the restroom Offer food or drink (if patient can tolerate)
Provide support/validation of the situation	"I would be upset too" "Let's figure this out together"
Providing step-by-step expectations	"Here is what you can expect during your visit today"
Offering patient choices or options	Offering oral anxiolytics Discuss physical restraint removal (if applicable)

respiratory depression than benzodiazepines.[2,5–7] Droperidol 5–10 mg IM as monotherapy will safely quiet most disruptive patients with moderate agitation in 5–15 minutes. Antipsychotics are the preferred treatment of agitation thought to be due to psychiatric disease, medical delirium, or dementia.

Despite decades of widespread use with an excellent record of safety, in 2001 the US Food and Drug Administration (FDA) issued a "black box" warning on droperidol for the potential of serious proarrhythmic effects associated with prolongation of the QT interval. The suspicious circumstances surrounding this labeling have been well-reported; however, the black box led to droperidol being unavailable in most US hospitals for many years.[8] Fortunately, droperidol returned to availability in 2019, and a plenitude of data attests to its safety when used in usual doses for a variety of indications, including ED-based treatment of agitation.[9–13] The American College of Emergency Physicians recommends that "physicians and out-of-hospital personnel continue to use droperidol at even higher doses, starting initially at 5 to 10 mg intramuscularly or intravenously given studied doses up to 20 mg, regardless of initial monitoring capability or EKG."[10]

Midazolam is the intramuscular benzodiazepine of choice for any indication, when speed and efficacy are of consequence, because midazolam has far more reliable absorption by the IM route than lorazepam and certainly diazepam, which should not be used IM. The dose of IM midazolam when used as monotherapy in the treatment of agitation in normal-sized non-elderly adults is 2–10 mg; however, doses >2 mg and especially ≥5 mg can cause respiratory depression, especially in the presence of other risk factors for respiratory depression such as alcohol intoxication, obesity, or obstructive sleep apnea. Benzodiazepines are the first-line treatment for agitation thought to be due to alcohol (or benzodiazepine) withdrawal or stimulant toxicity.

A combination of droperidol and midazolam will provide safe, effective, rapid sedation of nearly all agitated patients. For undifferentiated agitation, excellent results will usually be achieved with 5–10 mg droperidol, depending on patient size and degree of agitation, mixed with 2–5 mg mg midazolam.[14,15] If droperidol is not available or if QT interval is a particular concern, olanzapine is an effective alternative, with a 50% increase in dose. The FDA has expressed concern around the use of olanzapine with benzodiazepines; however, this concern is poorly evidence-supported.[2,16] Haloperidol is also an appropriate substitute, again at 50% higher dose than would be used for droperidol. See Figure 2.1.

It is common at many centers to add 25–50 mg diphenhydramine to sedation cocktails; however, this does not improve efficacy and is associated with significantly increased length of stay, oxygen desaturation, and use of physical restraints.[17] An antimuscarinic should be administered when indicated for extrapyramidal symptoms but not added routinely to calming medications.

Continuous monitoring of ventilation should be considered in any patient who receives sedating medications, based on an assessment of risk to develop respiratory depression. Pulse oximetry reliably detects hypoventilation in patients who are breathing room air; patients who require supplemental oxygen and are at risk for respiratory depression should be monitored with continuous end-tidal capnography.[18] Physical restraints should rarely be needed in this group; see the discussion of physical restraints below.

For many *disruptive without danger* patients, targeted history and physical exam provides sufficient confidence that an uneventful discharge will follow a period of restful metabolism, and in many cases no ancillary studies are indicated beyond a capillary blood glucose. Frequent reassessments and a repeat history and physical exam once the patient has

Choice of Initial Calming Medications in the Emergency Department

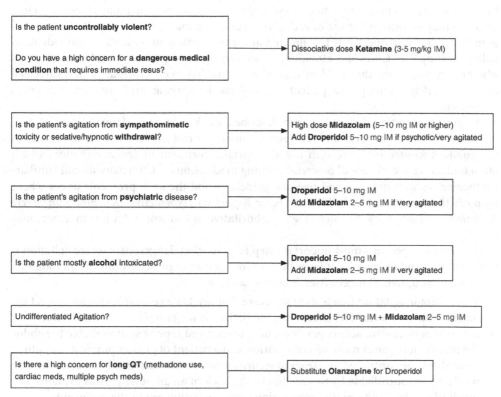

Is the patient **uncontrollably violent**? Do you have a high concern for a **dangerous medical condition** that requires immediate resus?	▶ Dissociative dose **Ketamine** (3–5 mg/kg IM)
Is the patient's agitation from **sympathomimetic** toxicity or sedative/hypnotic **withdrawal**?	▶ High dose **Midazolam** (5–10 mg IM or higher) Add **Droperidol** 5–10 mg IM if psychotic/very agitated
Is the patient's agitation from **psychiatric** disease?	▶ **Droperidol** 5–10 mg IM Add **Midazolam** 2–5 mg IM if very agitated
Is the patient mostly **alcohol** intoxicated?	▶ **Droperidol** 5–10 mg IM Add **Midazolam** 2–5 mg IM if very agitated
Undifferentiated Agitation?	▶ **Droperidol** 5–10 mg IM + **Midazolam** 2–5 mg IM
Is there a high concern for **long QT** (methadone use, cardiac meds, multiple psych meds)	▶ Substitute **Olanzapine** for Droperidol

If **haloperidol** or **olanzapine** substituted for droperidol, increase dose by ~50%

Figure 2.1 Choice of initial calming medication in the Emergency Department

emerged from sedation, including a discussion around unhealthy substance use and possible initiation of treatment of any substance-use disorders, completes the emergency management of the moderately agitated patient.

Dangerously Severe Agitation

Dangerously severe agitation is an uncommon but cardinal emergency presentation requiring the full scope of the emergency physician's skillset. The dangerously agitated patient presents immediate danger: danger to themself and others from uncontrolled psychomotor agitation, and the danger from one or more life threats that may be either its cause or consequence. Dangerously severe agitation is not only more serious in magnitude; the potential for danger demands a strategy that is different in kind than the measured, stepwise approach used in the management of mild or moderate agitation.

Dangerous agitation, especially in the prehospital domain, has become a matter of public scrutiny, in particular, agitation that involves law enforcement. The terms *excited delirium* and *agitated delirium* have been problematic since their inception, as they describe a syndrome but do not have diagnostic criteria, and many authors question whether excited delirium is a diagnostic entity at all. Making the "diagnosis" of excited delirium may distract clinicians from underlying conditions that require specific treatments. Furthermore, voices from across the spectrum of medicine, law, and public discourse warn that a label of excited delirium may encourage the use of excessive force in the management of agitation, or may even be applied retrospectively to validate improper handling of patients or individuals in police custody.[19-22] Clinicians attending to severely agitated patients should not focus on whether an imaginary threshold of excited delirium has been crossed; rather, direct all efforts to safely calming the patient, as well as identifying and treating dangerous conditions.

Hypersympathetic delirium has been described and known to be dangerous for centuries, however, and prehospital and emergency clinicians must not let social controversies in the public discourse interfere with the appropriate treatment of severe agitation, which often indicates the early use of powerful calming medications.[23] Clinicians should familiarize themselves with national and regional guidelines and the local protocols under whose auspices they practice; the *ACEP Task Force Report on Hyperactive Delirium with Severe Agitation in Emergency Settings* is an authoritative document relevant to emergency care.[24,25]

The first and perhaps most important step in managing dangerously severe agitation is to recognize it and distinguish it from the far more common presentations of agitation that are merely disruptive. Danger arises from two sources:

1. Psychomotor agitation that is itself so severe that available resources cannot protect the patient and others from its effects; i.e., the patient is *uncontrollably violent*. What constitutes uncontrollable depends on the number and type of staff available to subdue the patient; it requires more severe agitation and a patient of greater physical strength to be unable to be controlled by a team of security guards in an emergency department than would be uncontrollable by two medics in the back of an ambulance; this explains why much of the data and opinion concerning severe agitation are in the prehospital literature. Managing a severely agitated patient in a space-limited urban ED may be riskier than in more open suburban or rural settings, which would appropriately tilt management of agitation as "uncontrollable" when the same patient could otherwise be handled using a slower, stepwise approach.

2. When agitation accompanies a *high concern for an immediately dangerous condition* requiring prompt treatment that cannot be rendered due to the patient's resistance. The classic example is the agitated polytrauma patient with evidence of potentially life-threatening injury; the threshold to initiate prompt, assertive treatment of agitation (often by rapid sequence intubation and intubation) is appropriately low, so that dangerous injuries can be quickly identified and managed. The same paradigm applies to the patient struggling to breathe while ripping off their facemask, where agitation is often the consequence of hypoxia, or the stimulant-intoxicated patient thrashing about the stretcher with a temperature of 41°C.

In both of these circumstances – the uncontrollably violent patient, and the patient with high concern for a dangerous condition – the priority is effectively treating agitation as rapidly as feasible, so that the hazards arising from agitation are diminished, and so that the focus of care can quickly shift from control to resuscitation.

Uncontrollable violence is manifest and easily recognized; dangerous medical conditions underlying or accompanying agitation may be hidden, and often clinical experience and careful judgment are required to differentiate the dangerously agitated patient from the simply intoxicated patient who needs only to sleep it off. The degree of agitation is the first clue: dangerously agitated patients are often not just yelling and shouting, they are *thrashing*, held down and struggling to break free despite futility or pain, seemingly without tiring. The delirious patient potentially harboring a dangerous condition is often not just angry, but *incoherent* and un-engageable, unable to participate in conversation, their cognition or level of consciousness *fluctuating* in a way that you don't see in the merely drunk. *Vital signs* as usual may offer important guidance; however, vitals may be unobtainable, and if a team of security guards is required to hold down the patient to get vitals, that patient is more likely to be harboring a dangerous agitation and it may be prudent to proceed according to principles for managing severe, dangerous agitation prior to obtaining a full set of vital signs.

Once dangerously severe agitation has been recognized, the first step in management is to assemble adequate force to safely subdue the patient. Ideally, this would be five people – one for each limb and one for the head – which does not include the clinician attending the patient or the nurse preparing and administering medications. Personnel resources available to manage agitation vary across settings; however, readiness can be improved by developing an agitation code response team that triggers appropriate resources to bedside and protocolized workflows to optimize agitation care.[26]

When adequate force has allowed for the severely agitated patient to be safely approached, face mask oxygen covering the mouth and nose should be applied to the patient, with the strings tightened so that the mask is closely affixed to the face. Early use of face mask oxygen empirically treats hypoxia, a critical cause of agitation, and is especially valuable to control spitting in the agitated patient, whose mouth and nose may be covered by a gloved hand, which is an asphyxiation risk.[25]

At this stage, the clinician should deliberately identify and relieve dangerous restraint holds, which are often used to control a violent patient and include compression of the neck or chest/back, straightjackets, and especially the hog tie or hobble position where the prone patient's hands are bound to their ankles; this position is strongly associated with death in custody and should never be used.[27,28]

Once dangerously severe agitation has been identified, the patient has been apprehended by adequate force, face mask oxygen has been applied, and dangerous restraint holds relieved, the patient's agitation should be treated with maximally effective calming medications. Unless intravenous access that is known to be functioning is already in place, calming medications should be delivered by the intramuscular route.[22] Although it is routine in some centers to attempt IV access on an agitated patient being held down, this strategy needlessly subjects staff to the risk of needlestick and may delay treatment, as starting a line on a diaphoretic, writhing patient often requires multiple attempts. IM treatment is fast, effective, and may be administered through the clothing.[29,30]

The pharmacologic approach to the treatment of dangerously severe agitation differs importantly compared to the management of patients who are merely disruptive. The prime concern in calming moderately agitated patients is to minimize the chance of adverse medication effects, at the cost of slower effectiveness and the possible need for repeat dosing. Conversely, the priority in managing dangerously agitated patients is rapid calming, so that dangerous violence can be contained and dangerous conditions can be identified and addressed. Deep sedation and its consequences (mainly respiratory depression, which is readily redressed) are accepted and anticipated in exchange for immediate, effective agitation treatment. Furthermore, the need to intubate the dangerously agitated patient in order to achieve control, or as a consequence of achieving control through the proper use of maximally effective medications, is not an error or an adverse event; airway management is a predictable, appropriate, and sometimes necessary part of the treatment of severe agitation.

Because the priority in the management of dangerously severe agitation is maximally rapid and effective treatment, in a single intramuscular shot, the sedative of choice is dissociative-dose ketamine. Ketamine, when administered in a dose of 3–5 mg/kg, has excellent IM pharmacokinetics and renders nearly every patient calm, regardless of the underlying physiology or toxicology, in less than 5 minutes, while airway, breathing, and circulation are *usually* maintained.

A theoretical objection to the use of dissociative-dose ketamine for agitation is ketamine's catecholaminergic effects when given to calm patients for procedural sedation; however, vital signs of severely agitated, hyperdynamic patients will normalize when treated with ketamine.[31,32] Other concerns, such as worsening of intracranial or intraocular pressure or exacerbation of underlying psychiatric disease, have not been borne out in published experience and trial data.[33-37] Although some series demonstrate high rates of intubation of agitated patients treated with ketamine, this in many cases represents clinician discomfort with dissociation rather than the need for intubation.[38] Furthermore, when airway management is necessary, intubation of dangerously agitated patients is proper, safety-preserving care.[4,39] The use of ketamine to treat undifferentiated severe agitation has been demonstrated to be safe and effective across a wide range of prehospital and emergency department studies.[40-50] An alternative to ketamine in the treatment of dangerously severe agitation is the combination of a high-dose benzodiazepine and antipsychotic, such as ≥10 mg IM midazolam and ≥10 mg IM droperidol.

Non-intubated patients treated with dissociative dose ketamine or high-dose benzodiazepines require resuscitation-level care, including procedural sedation monitoring and full airway setup with vigilant attention to ventilation and an airway-capable clinician continuously available. Apart from the risk of cardiorespiratory compromise assumed by the use of powerful sedatives, low-ratio, critical care nursing is appropriate to manage the pace of treatment required to manage patients with dangerously severe agitation.

It is usual practice in many centers to apply tight physical restraints to agitated patients prior to treating agitation with medications, or after medications have been administered, as the patient calms. The emphasis on physical restraint, rather than using medications to calm a moderately or severely agitated patient, is misdirected, and is a dangerous, punitive, discriminatory tradition worthy of condemnation. The agitated patient who is restrained but not calmed remains a threat to himself (if not others) through ongoing struggle; the time spent applying restraints is therefore time wasted against effective treatment that will abridge the risks directly arising from agitation and facilitate the identification and treatment of underlying dangerous conditions. Furthermore, physical restraints have been used as "punishment" for behaviors that agitated patients (many of whom are delirious) have directed toward clinicians and others, and constitute perhaps unintentional but nevertheless unacceptable acts of retribution that evidence suggests are affected by racial or cultural bias.[51-54]

Once adequate force has subdued the patient, all efforts should be directed at the treatment of agitation with medications. As the patient calms, the team, instead of moving to apply physical restraints, should remain in position until the patient calms.

The persistence or return of agitation indicates the need for additional treatment, not physical restraints.

If physical restraints are used, they should be applied for the shortest duration possible based on frequent reassessment, as treatment of agitation is ongoing. Documentation according to a protocolized note or flowsheet should clearly describe and support why safety could not be maintained by alternatives.

As the patient calms, the clinician's focus pivots from control to resuscitation. The patient should be appropriately positioned on the bed, with the head of the bed elevated, and any tight restraints should be loosened or removed. Continuous cardiorespiratory monitoring should be instituted as early as feasible and include room air saturation; if supplemental oxygen is required in the non-intubated patient at risk for respiratory depression, ventilation should be monitored with continuous waveform capnography. Core temperature and capillary blood glucose are essential measurements in this group at the outset of care. Resuscitative vascular access should be obtained, and nearly all severely agitated patients will benefit from crystalloid volume so an empiric bolus is usually appropriate.

Once initial resuscitative maneuvers have been performed, attention shifts to identifying and treating the principle dangerous causes and effects of severe agitation. The most immediately dangerous conditions associated with severe agitation include hypoxia, hyperthermia, hypoglycemia, and hypoperfusion from either volume loss or hemorrhage. Hyperkalemia and acidemia should be excluded in all patients, with early consideration to evaluate for intracranial hemorrhage and central nervous system (CNS) infection. The remainder of the differential diagnosis for severe agitation is wide and includes alcohol or other sedative withdrawal, serotonin syndrome, thyrotoxicosis, seizure or postictal state, sepsis, and metabolic encephalopathies such as hyperammonemia.

Rhabdomyolysis and trauma are common dangerous consequences of severe agitation and routine measurement of creatinine kinase is indicated, as is a careful examination for evidence of occult trauma. It is appropriate to have a low threshold to perform imaging, especially of the brain, as these patients are at high risk for injury and are often poorly evaluable for some hours after pharmacologic treatment of agitation.

A summary of the initial management of dangerously severe agitation is presented in Table 2.2.

Vignette Conclusion

It is quickly recognized that this patient, who is incoherent and struggling to break free of overwhelming force, is dangerously agitated. Face mask oxygen is applied to the patient's mouth and nose as the forearm of one of the police officers, which was compressing the patient's chest, is repositioned. Ketamine (500 mg) is administered intramuscularly through the patient's jeans. As the patient calms, he is attached to a monitor, repositioned in bed, and the head of the bed is elevated. After 5 minutes the patient is fully dissociated so the team releases the patient, clothing is quickly cut and removed, and two large-bore IVs are established. The physician requests a 1-liter bolus of lactated ringers and a full set of vitals including rectal temperature and fingerstick, while performing a careful head to toe exam, which shows dry mucous membranes, nystagmus, and subtle bruising of the left flank. Initial workup shows a core temperature of 41°C and creatinine kinase > 30,000; imaging demonstrates two rib fractures and a small subdural hemorrhage. Appropriate treatments are initiated and the patient requires several doses of intravenous lorazepam in the ED.

Table 2.2 Initial Management of Dangerously Severe Agitation

- Assemble adequate force to safely approach and subdue the patient
- Apply face mask oxygen to cover the mouth and nose
- Relieve restraint holds that compress the neck, chest, or back (especially the hog tie)
- Administer maximally effective calming medication intramuscularly, e.g., ketamine 5 mg/kg IM
- Loosen any tight restraints applied
- Position the patient safely in bed, head of bed ≥30°
- Vital signs including core temperature, glucose, and room air saturation
- Continuous cardiorespiratory monitoring, including capnography if supplemental oxygen
- Vascular access and crystalloid bolus
- Exclude or treat hypoxia, hyperthermia, hypoglycemia, hypoperfusion, hyperkalemia, acidemia, and rhabdomyolysis
- Consider ancillary testing to exclude trauma (especially intracranial hemorrhage), and CNS infection
- Gather needed information to identify other causes and effects of severe agitation

Several hours after admission to the trauma service, the patient's mental status clears and he reports that everything was fine until he snorted "something, I don't even know what" at the club. He is discharged 2 days later in good condition.

Pro-Tips

- Distinguishing the merely disruptive patient from the dangerously agitated patient may be challenging but is the critical decision point for the emergency clinician.
- Disruptive patients who are not calmed with verbal de-escalation are managed with an emphasis on medication safety, using a titratable antipsychotic, benzodiazepine, or combination.
- Dangerously agitated patients require the focus of care be on immediate control, so that attention can pivot to identification and treatment of dangerous conditions.
- The initial management of the dangerously agitated patient begins with an appropriately trained and resourced team applying safe restraint holds, face mask oxygen, and the prompt intramuscular administration of a medication or medications that will reliably calm the patient, such as dissociative-dose ketamine.
- Once the patient has calmed, resuscitation begins in customary fashion with the establishment of intravenous access and cardiopulmonary monitoring, with attention to life threats such as hyperthermia, hypoxia, hypovolemia, and serious injuries.

References

1. Peisah C, Chan DK, McKay R, Kurrle SE, Reutens SG. Practical guidelines for the acute emergency sedation of the severely agitated older patient. *Internal Med J*. 2011;41(9):651–657.

2. Klein LR, Driver BE, Miner JR, Martel ML, Hessel M, Collins JD, Horton GB, Fagerstrom E, Satpathy R, Cole JB. Intramuscular midazolam, olanzapine, ziprasidone, or haloperidol for treating acute

agitation in the emergency department. *Ann Emerg Med.* 2018;72(4):374–385.

3. Wilson MP, Pepper D, Currier GW, Holloman Jr GH, Feifel D. The psychopharmacology of agitation: consensus statement of the American Association for Emergency Pyschiatry project beta workshop. *West J Emerg Med.* 2012;13(1):26–34. PMID: 22461918.

4. Strayer R. Jon Cole on Ketamine for Agitation. *Emergency Medicine Updates.* Available from: https://emupdates.com/jon-cole-on-ketamine-for-agitation (accessed April 23, 2022).

5. Isbister GK, Calver LA, Page CB, Stokes B, Bryant JL, Downes MA. Randomized controlled trial of intramuscular droperidol versus midazolam for violence and acute behavioral disturbance: the DORM study. *Ann Emerg Med.* 2010;56(4):392–401.

6. Knott JC, Taylor DM, Castle DJ. Randomized clinical trial comparing intravenous midazolam and droperidol for sedation of the acutely agitated patient in the emergency department. *Ann Emerg Med.* 2006;47(1):61–67.

7. Martel M, Sterzinger A, Miner J, Clinton J, Biros M. Management of acute undifferentiated agitation in the emergency department: a randomized double-blind trial of droperidol, ziprasidone, and midazolam. *Acad Emerg Med.* 2005;12 (12):1167–1172.

8. Lenzer J, Solomon RC. The droperidol dilemma: is the FDA's black box warning necessary? *ACEP News.* 2002;3(8).

9. Hernández-Rodríguez L, Bellolio F, Cabrera D, Mattson AE, VanMeter D, Grush AE, Silva LJE. Prospective real-time evaluation of the QTc interval variation after low-dose droperidol among emergency department patients. *Am J Emerg Med.* 2022;52: 212–219.

10. American College of Emergency Physicians. Policy statements. *Ann Emerg Med.* 2021;77(6):e127–e133.

11. Cole JB, Lee SC, Martel ML, Smith SW, Biros MH, Miner JR. The incidence of QT prolongation and torsades des pointes in patients receiving droperidol in an urban emergency department. *West J Emerg Med.* 2020;21(4):728–736.

12. Gaw CM, Cabrera D, Bellolio F, Mattson AE, Lohse CM, Jeffery MM. Effectiveness and safety of droperidol in a United States emergency department. *Am J Emerg Med.* 2020;38(7):1310–1314.

13. Calver L, Page CB, Downes MA, Chan B, Kinnear F, Wheatley L, Spain D, Isbister GK. The safety and effectiveness of droperidol for sedation of acute behavioral disturbance in the emergency department. *Ann Emerg Med.* 2015;66(3):230–238.

14. Yap CY, Taylor DM, Knott JC, Taylor SE, Phillips GA, Karro J, Chan EW, Kong DC, Castle DJ. Intravenous midazolam–droperidol combination, droperidol or olanzapine monotherapy for methamphetamine-related acute agitation: subgroup analysis of a randomized controlled trial. *Addiction.* 2017;112 (7):1262–1269.

15. Taylor DM, Yap CY, Knott JC, Taylor SE, Phillips GA, Karro J, Chan EW, Kong DC, Castle DJ. Midazolam–droperidol, droperidol, or olanzapine for acute agitation: a randomized clinical trial. *Ann Emerg Med.* 2017;69(3):318–326.

16. Westefer L, Faust J. Olanzapine + Benzodiazepines – What Is the FDA Warning About? *FOAMcast.* Available from: https://foamcast.org/2019/10/29/olanzapine-benzodiazepines-what-is-the-fda-warning-about (accessed April 12, 2022).

17. Jeffers T, Darling B, Edwards C, Vadiei N. Efficacy of combination haloperidol, lorazepam, and diphenhydramine vs. combination haloperidol and lorazepam in the treatment of acute agitation: a multicenter retrospective cohort study. *J Emerg Med.* 2022;62(4):516–523.

18. Witting MD, Hsu S, Granja CA. The sensitivity of room-air pulse oximetry in the detection of hypercapnia. *Am J Emerg Med.* 2005;23(4):497–500.

19. Strömmer EM, Leith W, Zeegers MP, Freeman MD. The role of restraint in fatal excited delirium: a research synthesis and pooled analysis. *Forensic Sci Med Pathol.* 2020;16(4):680–692.

20. Fiscella K, Pinals DA, Shields CG. "Excited delirium," erroneous concepts, dehumanizing language, false narratives, and threat to Black lives. *Acad Emerg Med.* 2022;29(7):911–913.

21. Saadi A, Naples-Mitchell J, da Silva Bhatia B, Heisler M. End the use of "excited delirium" as a cause of death in police custody. *Lancet.* 2022;399(10329):1028–1030.

22. Storey ML. Explaining the unexplainable: excited delirium syndrome and its impact on the objective reasonableness standard for allegations of excessive force. *St Louis Univ Law J.* 2012;56(2):10.

23. Kraines SH. Bell's mania. *Am J Psychiatry.* 1934;91(1):29–40.

24. ACEP Hyperactive Delirium Task Force. ACEP Task Force Report on Hyperactive Delirium with Severe Agitation in Emergency Settings. American College of Emergency Physicians; 2021. www.acep.org/globalassets/new-pdfs/education/acep-task-force-report-on-hyperactive-delirium-final.pdf (accessed April 28, 2022).

25. Kupas DF, Wydro GC, Tan DK, Kamin R, Harrell IV AJ, Wang A. Clinical care and restraint of agitated or combative patients by emergency medical services practitioners. *Prehosp Emerg Care.* 2021;25(5):721–723.

26. Wong AH, Ray JM, Cramer LD, Brashear TK, Eixenberger C, McVaney C, Haggan J, Sevilla M, Costa DS, Parwani V, Ulrich A. Design and implementation of an agitation code response team in the emergency department. *Ann Emerg Med.* 2022;79(5):453–464.

27. Stratton SJ, Rogers C, Green K. Sudden death in individuals in hobble restraints during paramedic transport. *Ann Emerg Med.* 1995;25(5):710–712.

28. Strömmer EM, Leith W, Zeegers MP, Freeman MD. The role of restraint in fatal excited delirium: a research synthesis and pooled analysis. *Forensic Sci Med Pathol.* 2020;16(4):680–692.

29. Khawaja RA, Sikandar R, Qureshi R, Jareno RJ. Routine skin preparation with 70% isopropyl alcohol swab: is it necessary before an injection? Quasi study. *J Liaquat Uni Med Health Sci.* 2013;12(02):109–114.

30. Fleming DR, Jacober SJ, Vandenberg MA, Fitzgerald JT, Grunberger G. The safety of injecting insulin through clothing. *Diabetes Care.* 1997;20(3):244–247.

31. Scheppke KA, Braghiroli J, Shalaby M, Chait R. Prehospital use of IM ketamine for sedation of violent and agitated patients. *West J Emerg Med.* 2014;15(7):736–741.

32. Hopper AB, Vilke GM, Castillo EM, Campillo A, Davie T, Wilson MP. Ketamine use for acute agitation in the emergency department. *J Emerg Med.* 2015;48(6):712–719.

33. Green SM, Andolfatto G, Krauss BS. Ketamine and intracranial pressure: no contraindication except hydrocephalus. *Ann Emerg Med.* 2015;65(1):52–54.

34. Drayna PC, Estrada C, Wang W, Saville BR, Arnold DH. Ketamine sedation is not associated with clinically meaningful elevation of intraocular pressure. *Am J Emerg Med.* 2012;30(7):1215–1218.

35. Halstead SM, Deakyne SJ, Bajaj L, Enzenauer R, Roosevelt GE. The effect of ketamine on intraocular pressure in pediatric patients during procedural sedation. *Acad Emerg Med.* 2012;19(10):1145–1150.

36. Le Cong M, Humble I. A ketamine protocol and intubation rates for psychiatric air medical retrieval. *Air Med J.* 2015 Nov 1;34(6):357–9.

37. Swaminathan A. Is Ketamine Contraindicated in Patients with Psychiatric Disorders? *RebelEM.* Available from: https://rebelem.com/is-ketamine-contraindicated-in-patients-with-psychiatric-disorders (accessed April 23, 2022).

38. Cole JB, Moore JC, Nystrom PC, Orozco BS, Stellpflug SJ, Kornas RL, Fryza BJ, Steinberg LW, O'Brien-Lambert A, Bache-Wiig P, Engebretsen KM. A prospective study of ketamine versus haloperidol for severe prehospital agitation. *Clin Toxicol.* 2016;54(7):556–562.

39. Olives TD, Nystrom PC, Cole JB, Dodd KW, Ho JD. Intubation of

profoundly agitated patients treated with prehospital ketamine. *Prehosp Disaster Med*. 2016;31(6):593–602.

40. Lin J, Figuerado Y, Montgomery A, Lee J, Cannis M, Norton VC, Calvo R, Sikand H. Efficacy of ketamine for initial control of acute agitation in the emergency department: a randomized study. *Am J Emerg Med*. 2021;44:306–311.

41. Mo H, Campbell MJ, Fertel BS, Lam SW, Wells EJ, Casserly E, Meldon SW. Ketamine safety and use in the emergency department for pain and agitation/delirium: a health system experience. *West J Emerg Med*. 2020;21(2):272–281.

42. Barbic D, Andolfatto G, Grunau B, Scheuermeyer FX, Macewan B, Qian H, Wong H, Barbic SP, Honer WG. Rapid agitation control with ketamine in the emergency department: a blinded, randomized controlled trial. *Ann Emerg Med*. 2021;78(6):788–795.

43. Riddell J, Tran A, Bengiamin R, Hendey GW, Armenian P. Ketamine as a first-line treatment for severely agitated emergency department patients. *Am J Emerg Med*. 2017;35(7):1000–1004.

44. Friedman MS, Saloum D, Haaland A, Drapkin J, Likourezos A, Strayer RJ. Description of adverse events in a cohort of dance festival attendees with stimulant-induced severe agitation treated with dissociative-dose ketamine. *Prehosp Emerg Care*. 2021;25(6):761–767.

45. Heydari F, Gholamian A, Zamani M, Majidinejad S. Effect of intramuscular ketamine versus haloperidol on short-term control of severe agitated patients in emergency department; a randomized clinical trial. *Bull Emerg Trauma*. 2018;6 (4):292–299.

46. Gangathimmaiah V, Le Cong M, Wilson M, Hooper K, Perry A, Burman L, Puckeridge N, Maguire BJ. Ketamine sedation for patients with acute behavioral disturbance during aeromedical retrieval: a retrospective chart review. *Air Med J*. 2017;36(6):311–314.

47. Parsch CS, Boonstra A, Teubner D, Emmerton W, McKenny B, Ellis DY.

Ketamine reduces the need for intubation in patients with acute severe mental illness and agitation requiring transport to definitive care: an observational study. *Emerg Med Australas*. 2017;29(3):291–296.

48. Isoardi KZ, Parker LE, Page CB, Humphreys MA, Harris K, Rashford S, Isbister GK. Ketamine as a rescue treatment for severe acute behavioural disturbance: a prospective prehospital study. *Emerg Med Australas*. 2021;33(4):610–614.

49. Bernard S, Roggenkamp R, Delorenzo A, Stephenson M, Smith K, Ketamine in Severely Agitated Patients Study Investigators, Augello M, Buntine P, Costa S, Gaeboc M, Graudins A. Use of intramuscular ketamine by paramedics in the management of severely agitated patients. *Emerg Med Australas*. 2021;33 (5):875–882.

50. Isbister GK, Calver LA, Downes MA, Page CB. Ketamine as rescue treatment for difficult-to-sedate severe acute behavioral disturbance in the emergency department. *Ann Emerg Med*. 2016;67 (5):581–587.

51. Nash KA, Tolliver DG, Taylor RA, Calhoun AJ, Auerbach MA, Venkatesh AK, Wong AH. Racial and ethnic disparities in physical restraint use for pediatric patients in the emergency department. *JAMA Pediatr*. 2021;175(12):1283–1285.

52. Wong AH, Taylor RA, Ray JM, Bernstein SL. Physical restraint use in adult patients presenting to a general emergency department. *Ann Emerg Med*. 2019;73 (2):183–192.

53. Schnitzer K, Merideth F, Macias-Konstantopoulos W, Hayden D, Shtasel D, Bird S. Disparities in care: the role of race on the utilization of physical restraints in the emergency setting. *Acad Emerg Med*. 2020;27(10):943–950.

54. Wong AH, Whitfill T, Ohuabunwa EC, Ray JM, Dziura JD, Bernstein SL, Taylor RA. Association of race/ethnicity and other demographic characteristics with use of physical restraints in the emergency department. *JAMA Network Open*. 2021;4 (1):e2035241.

Penetrating Trauma

Alejandro A. Palma, Doreen Agboh, and Devon Fiorino

Vignette 1

A 31-year-old male presents to a Level 1 Trauma Center via emergency medical services (EMS) with two gunshot wounds to his abdomen that occurred 20 minutes prior to arrival. Emergency medical services reports minimal blood loss. The patient has no known past medical history, past surgical history, or allergies, and takes no medications. He does not know his last tetanus vaccination. Upon arrival to the Emergency Department (ED), the patient is alert and in mild distress. Vitals include: BP 134/87, P 95, RR 21, O_2 99% on room air.

Primary survey is notable for airway intact, bilateral breath sounds, 2+ bilateral femoral pulses, Glasgow Coma Score (GCS) 15. Focused Assessment with Sonography in Trauma (FAST) is positive in the right upper quadrant. Chest x-ray has no cardiopulmonary abnormality. The secondary exam is notable for two gunshot wounds, one to his left upper quadrant, and one to his left mid abdomen.

- What resuscitation is appropriate for this patient?
- What imaging is appropriate for this patient?

Vignette 2

A 24-year-old male arrives via EMS to a Level 1 Trauma Center after sustaining a gunshot wound to his right thigh after an altercation at a bar. Per EMS, the patient lost a significant amount of blood at the scene. Emergency medical services placed a tourniquet to the upper right thigh; however, the bleeding is not well controlled. Upon arrival to the ED, the patient appears diaphoretic, is minimally responsive, and is cool to the touch. Initial vital signs are: BP 62/44, HR 142, RR 28, O_2 sat 97% on room air.

Shortly after the primary and secondary survey, the patient has no palpable carotid pulse.

- What approach is most appropriate in cardiac arrest in the setting of penetrating trauma?
- How should clinicians assess and manage vascular and orthopedic trauma?

Introduction

In patients with penetrating trauma, emergency physicians play a critical role in the initiation of the algorithmic evaluation and management of injuries that are pivotal to limb salvage and function.[1] They must efficiently stabilize the critical patient, identify life-threatening injuries, and activate the resources and specialists the patient needs in a timely fashion.[2] Treating penetrating traumatic injuries requires considerable coordination between the ED and specialists.

Urban-based clinicians are disproportionately responsible for the care of adult and pediatric patients suffering from penetrating traumatic injuries. What follows are guiding principles of the approach to the trauma patient with penetrating trauma, not an exhaustive review of trauma care.

The Right Emergency Department

Part of providing excellent care is to facilitate care in the right facility. In Vignette 1, the patient had penetrating trauma to his abdomen. A patient with a high-risk penetrating injury such as this will require a Level 1 Trauma Center. A Level 1 Trauma Center serves as a primary center for EMS runs and as referral centers for community hospitals. These centers have 24-hour in-hospital access to general surgeons and specialists such as anesthesia, emergency medicine, neurosurgery, orthopedic surgery, radiology, plastic surgery, and maxillofacial surgery. These centers also evaluate and treat a minimum number of trauma patients annually, meaning that they are experts in traumatic resuscitations.[3] If a high-risk patient needs one of the above services and is initially evaluated at a community hospital, they should be transferred expeditiously to a Level 1 Trauma Center after initial stabilization without delaying for definitive imaging.

Team Structure

The correct team structure is critical to providing quality care. While different trauma centers will have different team members depending on the relative size of their departments, the team members are generally mixtures of general surgeons and emergency medicine physicians. An emergency medicine physician should be at the head of the bed to assess and provide an airway as necessary. Some centers may use an anesthesiologist as primary airway or as a backup. There should be two additional clinicians, one on either side of the patient. One clinician should perform the primary and secondary survey, while the other should provide assistance as needed. Both of these clinicians are the primary procedural clinicians if the patient should need procedures during the trauma activation. Finally, there should be a final clinician that stands at the foot of the bed to lead the activation.

A very important component of the team structure is nursing and tech support. An ideal team would have two nurses, one on either side of the patient, to obtain vitals and access. A third nurse should record the event and chart as the activation is ongoing. Having at least one technician is sufficient to obtain essential materials as the activation progresses and provide further assistance. Each member of the team should know their role. While this may happen automatically in an experienced team, the physician leading the team should verbally confirm the role of each member of the team.

Environmental Control

Evaluating trauma patients requires a large number of healthcare clinicians to congregate in one area. While these trauma evaluations can naturally become chaotic, physicians should establish as orderly an environment as possible. It is important to only include staff who are immediately necessary for the primary and secondary survey. Exclude police officers, family members, registration staff, media, etc. Urban ED resuscitation rooms frequently have a smaller footprint compared to non-urban hospitals. The clinician should consider the physical space when assigning team members to the trauma team and minimize the size of the team when appropriate. In a non-urban setting in which penetrating traumas are less frequent, clinicians can expect an inordinate number of spectators. It is critically important that the clinician in these settings controls the environment and removes the spectators. Controlling the environment in the trauma bay also necessitates that as few people speak as possible. All clinicians in the trauma bay should perform closed-loop communication. Resuscitation spaces in urban EDs are often quite small relative to their non-urban counterparts, so control of the space is paramount.

After the team has completed the initial assessment and stabilized the penetrating trauma patient, clinicians should employ chaplains, violence recovery programs, trauma-informed care teams, and other adjunctive services to address and consequently reduce the emotional trauma that patients experience as a result of their acute injuries and enforce positive coping strategies.[4] This also allows for safe discharge of patients as well as resources for outpatient assistance. Furthermore, it is important to debrief with all team members, especially after complex trauma cases.[4]

Primary Survey

The primary survey comprises the critical initial steps in traumatic resuscitations. The purpose of the primary survey is to rapidly assess the patient for life-threatening injuries. The well-known mnemonic is referred to as the ABCDEs: airway, breathing, circulation, disability, and exposure. It is important to adhere to this structure, as this order assesses for injuries in terms of what is most likely to cause mortality most rapidly: airway obstruction, respiratory failure, hemorrhagic shock, and neurologic injury. It is important to assess the patient in this order and pause the resuscitation whenever an abnormal finding is noted to intervene on the injury.

A: Airway

If the patient is able to speak with a normal voice, is tolerating secretions, and the physician has no concerns for airway obstruction, the airway is patent, often referred to as "clear." If the airway is not clear, the physician should establish an airway preferably via an endotracheal intubation. A laryngeal mask airway (LMA) is sufficient in select cases. Assess and treat for airway injuries while maintaining cervical spine precautions.

B: Breathing

The physician should auscultate for bilateral breath sounds. If the patient with penetrating trauma does not have bilateral breath sounds, consider a hemothorax or pneumothorax and place a chest tube.

C: Circulation

Circulation refers to adequate blood flow. Clinicians should assess circulation by palpating central pulses, most often bilateral femoral pulses. One important component of the circulation exam is assessing for obvious signs of bleeding, particularly in a hypotensive patient. If signs of bleeding are found, the physician should pause the resuscitation and address the bleeding. First, the clinician should provide direct pressure to the bleeding wound. If the patient is hypotensive or tachycardic in a penetrating trauma with concern for hemorrhagic shock, clinicians should start volume resuscitation using warm fluids with rapid infusion. Blood products are preferred over crystalloid fluid, but fluid is acceptable if blood is not available.[5]

D: Disability

Disability refers to a brief neurologic exam. Clinicians use the Glasgow Coma Scale (GCS) to assess disability. If the trauma patient has a GCS less than 8, physicians should strongly consider intubation for airway protection.

E: Exposure

Exposure is the final step of the primary survey. Completely remove the patient's clothes to assess for any additional injuries, then cover the patient with warm blankets.

Primary Survey Adjuncts

After completing the primary survey, clinicians should utilize primary survey adjuncts as necessary. These include the Focused Assessment with Sonography in Trauma (FAST) exam, a chest x-ray, and a pelvic x-ray.

FAST Exam

The FAST exam (Focused Assessment with Sonography in Trauma) comprises point-of-care ultrasound imaging of the substernal view of the cardiac window, the right upper quadrant, the left upper quadrant, and the pelvis to visualize free fluid. The extended version, entitled the E-FAST, allows the clinician to image lung fields to assess for pneumothorax and hemothorax. The FAST exam was initially validated for evaluating patients with blunt trauma. However, it has also proved useful for evaluating patients with penetrating trauma. In a review of eight observational studies that used FAST exams in penetrating trauma, the prevalence of a positive FAST exam ranged from 24.2% to 56.3%.[6] The specificity ranged from 94.1% to 100%, making this exam highly specific, but not sensitive (28%–100%).[6] A FAST exam is helpful for patients with penetrating injuries who are unstable because it helps the trauma surgeons better prioritize their initial approach in the trauma bay and the operating room.[6]

Chest X-Ray

A portable chest x-ray is a common adjunct during a trauma resuscitation. Certain radiology studies argue that a chest x-ray should always be done in penetrating traumas as intrathoracic injury cannot be ruled out based on history and physical exam alone in penetrating trauma.[7] Some experienced practitioners, however, do not routinely use chest x-rays in the acute setting. Some clinicians evaluating an unstable trauma patient prefer a lung ultrasound, because it takes less time than a chest x-ray and provides similar data. Deciding between the routine use of a chest x-ray versus a lung ultrasound as a primary survey adjunct depends on the comfort and ultrasound experience of the practitioner and only applies to unstable patients.

Pelvic X-Ray

While a pelvic x-ray is traditionally a routine part of blunt trauma evaluations, it is not a vital component of the primary survey when evaluating a patient with penetrating trauma unless there are specific signs and symptoms of bony pelvic injury on the history and exam.[8]

Secondary Survey

The secondary survey is a brief but thorough head-to-toe exam to assess for injuries not discovered in the primary exam. Clinicians should not attempt a secondary survey until the primary survey is completed and the patient has been adequately resuscitated. The secondary survey comprises obtaining history from the patient including allergies, medications, past medical history, last meal, and the events leading up to and related to the injury (AMPLE). The secondary survey also includes a head-to-toe exam including palpation of facial and head bony structure, pupillary exam, chest wall palpation, abdominal palpation, assessment of the stability of the pelvis, and obvious deformities to the extremities. Assess the skin for wounds at this time. Additionally, roll the patient to examine the back by palpating the cervical, thoracic, and lumbar spines, assessing for tenderness or step-offs. Examine both axilla and the perineum to exclude injuries to these areas. If there is concern for neurologic injury or bleeding, physicians should also perform a digital rectal exam to assess rectal tone and assess for gross blood.[9]

Concurrent Evaluation and Treatment

The evaluation of a trauma patient requires concurrent evaluation and treatment by multiple members of a team. While one physician conducts the primary and secondary exams, the nurses should obtain bilateral intravenous (IV) access. While patients with penetrating traumatic extremity injuries should be approached during the primary survey in the same stepwise fashion as all trauma patients, special care should be paid to the placement of their intravenous lines. Do not place resuscitative IV lines in the injured extremity.[1] This includes femoral vein access with a central line in the injured extremity, as arterial reconstruction may require grafting of the ipsilateral saphenous vein.[1]

When placing IVs, the nurses should also draw blood for labs. Routine trauma labs include complete blood count (CBC), comprehensive metabolic panel (CMP), prothrombin time (PT) and partial thromboplastin time (PTT), type & screen, alcohol blood level, and lactate.[10] While a urinalysis and urine toxicology panel are routine, they are only selectively useful. Clinicians could forgo the urinalysis and toxicology panel at their discretion.

As discussed above, each step in the primary survey may prompt concurrent treatment during the resuscitation. While some of these treatments have been discussed above, such as a chest tube or blood resuscitation, there are still others to consider. For example, some patients, such as those presenting with open fractures, will require the appropriate antibiotic early in the patient's clinical course and tetanus booster administration.[1]

Patients who are unstable with a positive finding on the primary or secondary survey should immediately be transported to the operating room (OR). Patients who are stable can proceed to imaging.

Utility of Computed Tomography

Determining the extent of injuries in a patient suffering from a penetrating traumatic injury typically involves the use of computed tomography (CT). Computed tomography scans help trauma surgeons determine which patients need laparotomies or other interventions and assist the surgeons in surgical planning. Various studies have demonstrated that the use of CT decreases the rate of unnecessary laparotomies in stable patients.[11]

The type of CT scan depends on the clinical scenario. It is difficult to predict the trajectory of penetrating wounds, often necessitating more extensive imaging than the physical exam may indicate. For example, a gunshot wound to the abdomen, such as the wound in Vignette 1, requires a CT of the chest, abdomen, and pelvis. Some clinicians may also extend this imaging to the neck. It is important to consider the mechanism of the injury. For example, some clinicians are more comfortable limiting the scope of imaging in patients with stab wounds in certain locations compared to those with gunshot sounds. For example, a stable patient who reports a stab wound to the lower abdomen may only receive a CT of the abdomen and pelvis because the trajectory of a knife is more predictable than that of a bullet. It is important to note that patients with stab wounds in the upper quadrants should still receive a CT of the chest to assess for diaphragmatic injury or injury to the cardiac box if in the left upper quadrant. Additional history, such as whether the patient fell after the initial penetrating injury and sustained head trauma, could prompt additional imaging such as a head and cervical spine CT. In all cases, clinicians should preferentially order CT angiography to assess for active extravasation.

Penetrating Neck Trauma

Penetrating injuries to the neck require specific interventions as they are at high risk for decompensation. Traditionally, clinicians evaluated penetrating neck trauma in terms of zones, defined as:

Zone 1: area between the clavicles and the cricoid cartilage[12]

Zone 2: area between the cricoid cartilage and the angle of the mandible[12]

Zone 3: Area between the angle of the mandible and the base of the skull[12]

However, more emergency physicians and trauma surgeons have started to adopt the "no zone approach." While some clinicians still use the zonal approach in stable patients without a hard sign, newer data demonstrate that the no zone approach is associated with better outcomes.[13] In the no zone approach, patients with penetrating trauma to the neck should be assessed for hard signs.[14]

'Hard signs include:

- Airway compromise
- Stridor
- Hoarseness
- Difficulty or pain with swallowing secretions
- Bubbling from the wound
- Subcutaneous emphysema
- Shock
- Pulsatile bleeding
- Audible bruit or palpable thrill
- Neurological deficits

Patients with hard signs should immediately go to the OR. Patients who do not have a hard sign can receive a CT scan.

Management for penetrating neck trauma depends on the patient's stability. If the patient does not have a hard sign but is unstable, the patient should be transported to the OR immediately for definitive management. As stated above, patients with a hard sign should also go immediately to the OR regardless of stability. Patients who are stable without hard signs can go for a CT scan. Clinicians should order a CT angiogram (CTA) of the neck instead of a CT with contrast. C-collars are not routinely indicated for these patients as the rate of cervical spine injury is low.[15] Pediatric penetrating neck trauma guidelines follow those for adults.[16]

Evaluating the Penetrating Extremity Trauma Patient

Penetrating extremity trauma has an increased risk of vascular injury as compared to blunt trauma.[17] In the hospital setting, gunshot wounds are the most common cause of penetrating extremity trauma, followed by stab wounds.[10] While the cause of death for a majority of these patients is exsanguination, these patients also have the potential for morbidity from vascular lesions, neurological deficits, fractures, and limb loss.[17,18] Subsequently, penetrating extremity trauma has the risk for wound infection and thromboembolism.[19]

The first step in evaluating patients with penetrating extremity trauma is to assess the patient using the foundational guidelines of the Advanced Trauma Life Support (ATLS) protocol with the primary and secondary survey described above.[18] Although severe penetrating extremity trauma may serve as a distractor, resuscitation is the top priority in all trauma patients.[1] Remember the ABCDEs as discussed.

There are certain portions of the physical exam that clinicians should be more mindful of in a patient presenting with an extremity wound from penetrating trauma. In particular, the clinician should take note to palpate for pulses and control active bleeding during the primary exam.[10] Signs of acute large-volume blood loss include pooling blood and soaked garments. The initial management for acute bleeding is to apply direct pressure to the wound. If pressure is ineffective in controlling acute hemorrhage, pack the wound or place hemostatic dressings to control the bleeding. In certain wounds, such as those with pulsatile bleeding that do not respond to direct pressure or packing, clinicians can use a figure-of-eight stitch as a useful adjunct. It is important to be cognizant of objects that may inflict injury to the individual packing the wound, such as fractured bones or retained foreign bodies such as bullets, glass, and debris.

If a patient continues to actively bleed despite the use of a hemostatic dressing on an extremity wound, the physician should use a tourniquet to control the bleeding. The proper placement is critical for effective hemorrhage control. For extremity trauma, the ability to control ongoing hemorrhage with the proximal vessel occlusion is a unique advantage as compared to penetrating torso injury.[17] Note that a tourniquet is not effective for wounds in the axilla, groin, or torso, as there is no proximal location for tourniquet placement. While tourniquets can cause neurovascular injuries such as nerve damage and limb loss, there is only a 5% overall complication rate of tourniquets that are applied correctly.[18] Prehospital tourniquet placement has been associated with the reversal of the incidence of shock and a decreased usage of blood product secondary to adequate hemorrhage control without an increased risk of major tourniquet-related complications.[20] Thus, clinicians should readily use tourniquets when available for proper management of hemorrhage control. Note that tourniquets should not be left on for more than 6 hours to prevent tissue damage.

Additionally, it is crucial to perform a neurovascular examination of all extremities early during the secondary survey, paying particular attention to peripheral pulses and absent neurological function.[1,17,18] Evaluate for bony, soft tissue, vascular, and neurologic injury.[17]

The presence of absent or diminished neurological function of an extremity mandates an urgent evaluation and management.[1]

Vascular Injury

As compared to patients with blunt trauma, patients with penetrating trauma are more likely to suffer from vascular injuries that require operative management.[20] When examining for signs of hard vascular injury, look for active pulsatile bleeding, a rapidly expanding hematoma, pallor, pulselessness, paresthesia, paralysis, or a pulsatile bruit/thrill.[1,18,21] In patients with hard signs of vascular injury, bleeding control is of critical importance and should be addressed as a component of the circulation portion of the primary exam.[18] Patients with hard signs of arterial injury should undergo operative repair as soon as possible.[22] Soft signs of vascular injury include non-pulsatile bleeding, a non-expanding hematoma, a prior history of arterial bleeding, and the proximity of the wound to an artery.[2,17,19,21]

In stable patients and those with soft signs of vascular injury, physicians should use imaging studies and additional testing modalities to assess the degree of injury present. The Ankle Brachial Index (ABI) is the first modality that physicians should employ to assess the extremity for vascular compromise. To perform this technique, measure the systolic blood pressure in the affected limb and divide it by the systolic blood pressure in the unaffected limb.[18] If the ABI is greater than 0.9, this suggests that there is no vascular injury, with a 99% negative predictive value.[18] Note that normal ABIs without soft or hard signs of vascular injury suggest that there is no vascular compromise.[19] In patients with isolated extremity injuries, physicians should observe these patients for signs of clinical decline and discharge home if they remain stable. However, if the ABI is less than 0.9, patients should undergo further evaluation to assess for vascular compromise in the injured limb.

While conventional contrast angiography remains the gold standard for assessing for and intervening on vascular injury, CTA can rapidly diagnose vascular injury with similar specificity and sensitivity and provides a rapid assessment for examining vascular injuries that are clinically relevant.[18,22] Furthermore, in patients with stabilized bleeding, pre-procedural imaging via CTA provides invaluable information on identifying the location and extent of the vascular injury for surgical planning and thereby plays a pivotal role in identifying vascular injuries.[21,22] Thus, CTA is the primary imaging modality for evaluating vascular injury in patients with an ABI <0.9.[17]

Orthopedic Injury

In patients with penetrating trauma, there are often simultaneous vascular and orthopedic injuries.[1] Thus, it is important to have an algorithmic approach to managing these concomitant injuries. The stabilization of closed fractures that require closed reduction and external fixation should take precedence over definitive vascular repair.[1,17] However, vascular repair should precede orthopedic repair of injuries that require open reduction and internal fixation.[1] Pulseless limbs require urgent provisional reduction prior to definitive surgical fixation. Additionally, patients that are being transferred should have provisional reductions prior to transfer. Administer broad-spectrum antibiotics such as a third-generation cephalosporin and an aminoglycoside for severely contaminated wounds.[2] As mentioned above, patients should also receive a tetanus vaccination if they are not up to date.

In patients with penetrating extremity injuries, primary amputations are a rare occurrence, as most injuries can be operatively repaired.[1] Amputations are reserved for extreme presentations by which the patient has sustained extreme damage to the limb or where the primary amputation is needed for the patient to survive. The decision to amputate a limb should not be made in the acute trauma setting.[1]

Compartment Syndrome

It is important to be able to identify compartment syndrome in the acute setting while the patient is still in the ED. Compartment syndrome is a surgical emergency that can lead to irreversible tissue loss if not intervened on in a timely fashion. It occurs when there is increased pressure within the osteofascial compartment that compromises blood flow to tissues within that compartment, leading to irreversible muscle and nerve damage.[1] Once the pressure in a compartment reaches >30 mmHg, the lymphatic drainage systems can no longer adequately drain the edematous tissue, causing resultant hypoxia that alters cellular enzymatic activity and ultimately leads to free radical production.[1] This ultimately leads to compromised tissue perfusion. A difference of ≤30 mmHg between the systolic arterial pressure and the compartment is diagnostic of compartment syndrome.[1] Pain, pallor, pulselessness, paralysis, poikilothermia, and pain on passive stretch are clinically diagnostic of compartment syndrome.[1,2,10] Patients may also have the loss of two-point discrimination.[10] The most common cause of compartment syndrome is a tibial plateau fracture. The definitive management of compartment syndrome is a decompressive fasciotomy performed by either orthopedic or general surgeons.[1] Wide incisions allow for the complete release of the constrained fascia.[2] These patients will need admission as well as definitive surgical repair. Note that in all patients with vascular injury from penetrating trauma, they should have outpatient follow-up 1–2 weeks after discharge to evaluate for pseudoaneurysms and arteriovenous fistulas.[17]

Approach to the Critically Ill Patient

Recognizing shock early in the trauma clinical setting is crucial in improving survival outcomes.[5] In the critical patient who demonstrates shock, it is essential to mobilize the trauma surgery service for definitive operative intervention and management.[18] In centers without a dedicated trauma service, clinicians must transfer these patients to the nearest Level 1 Trauma Center after initial stabilization. All unstable penetrating trauma patients who demonstrate worsening hemodynamic instability or acute changes in their exam warrant immediate operative management.[18] Additionally, if time warrants, document a neurologic examination so that any neurological changes postoperatively can be properly addressed.

In the acute trauma setting, patients in extremis can rapidly deteriorate to traumatic arrest. Hemorrhage is the most reversible cause of trauma arrest.[5,23] Thus, rapid blood replacement is key in patients with active hemorrhage. Additional management of bleeding focuses on preventing blood loss and maintaining blood circulation.[5] In the event of a traumatic cardiac arrest, chest compressions are critical in maintaining circulation and perfusion.[24] An emergency thoracotomy should be performed for patients that have witnessed traumatic arrests less than 15 minutes of pre-hospital cardiopulmonary resuscitation (CPR) following penetrating injury to the torso, less than 5 minutes of prehospital CPR in patients following penetrating injury to the neck or extremity, and patients in profound refractory shock per the Western Association for the Surgery of Trauma guidelines.[24] Clinicians should perform open cardiac massage to maximize perfusion to tissues.[24] Following Advanced Cardiac Life Support (ACLS) guidelines, physicians should give epinephrine and additional adjuncts when warranted. In the emergent thoracotomy setting, administer epinephrine via the intracardiac route. It is also important to assess for reversible causes of traumatic arrest such as hemothorax, pneumothorax, and cardiac tamponade and intervene on them in the acute setting. If return of spontaneous circulation (ROSC) is obtained, these patients will require definitive operative management. It is important to note that a thoracotomy should never be performed in a facility without definitive surgical intervention available. Resuscitative efforts should be withheld in cases of prolonged traumatic resuscitation or obvious signs of death.[24] While survival has steadily increased due to improvements in medical interventions, patients that present to the hospital as traumatic arrests patients have poor outcomes, with only 11.1% surviving to hospital discharge.[25]

Pediatric Trauma

For all pediatric trauma patients, EMS should prioritize transportation to a pediatric trauma center. While penetrating trauma is less common in children than adults, it is important to be cognizant of the anatomic and physiologic differences between children and adults when evaluating pediatric patients.[26] Children's airways are more anterior than adults and they have floppier epiglottises, which may make intubations more challenging.[26] In regards to thoracic injury, the spleen and liver are larger and more anterior in children.[26] Additionally, they have less subcutaneous fat; therefore, there is a high risk of solid organ injury in children. In the critically ill pediatric trauma patient, note that children are able to maintain hemodynamic stability despite large-volume blood loss due to differences in their physiology, thus changes in their vital signs may imply an impending traumatic arrest.[26] Children have open growth plates, thus limb length discrepancies are possible during wound healing for children that sustain orthopedic injuries.[26] Additionally, medication dosages and blood resuscitation should be weight-based in children. Broselow pediatric emergency tape is a helpful adjunct in quickly determining the appropriate dosages for pediatric trauma patients.

Vignette 1 Conclusion

This patient was brought to a Level 1 Trauma Center, an appropriate location for this patient. This patient is stable based on his vitals. His airway is intact, he has bilateral breath sounds, and his heart rate and blood pressure are within normal limits. He does not require resuscitation at this time. If he were tachycardic, the clinician should consider blood transfusion preferably or crystalloid if blood were unavailable. Additionally, the clinician should make note of the hemostasis of each gunshot wound, providing direct pressure, gauze, or a figure-of-eight suture as necessary.

This stable patient has a positive fast with known penetrating abdominal trauma. A CT abdomen/pelvis is necessary. A CTA is the preferred choice to assess for active extravasation. The patient should also receive a CTA chest as the trajectory of penetrating trauma is difficult to predict. If the patient reported headache, neck pain, back pain, or other concerning signs or symptoms, the physician should expand imaging to include CTA neck, CT head, and CT lumbar and CT thoracic spine.

Vignette 2 Conclusion

What Approach Should Be Taken in Traumatic Arrests in the Setting of Penetrating Trauma?

Given that the patient had a witnessed traumatic cardiac arrest, the team should perform an emergent thoracotomy in the trauma bay. Following ACLS guidelines, the team should perform cardiac massage and give intracardiac epinephrine. The aorta is cross-clamped (or manually compressed). The patient should also receive rapid volume resuscitation with the massive transfusion protocol. In the above vignette, an additional tourniquet placed above the right thigh gunshot wound controls the active bleeding. After two rounds of CPR, the patient obtains ROSC. The trauma surgery team takes the patient emergently to the OR to perform definitive management.

How Should Vascular and Orthopedic Trauma Be Assessed and Managed?

Given the active pulsatile bleeding noted on exam in this vignette, this patient demonstrates a hard sign of vascular injury. In the immediate interim, a tourniquet controls the bleeding. The team assessed for vascular compromise in a timely fashion during the primary survey and started active resuscitation. This patient will require urgent operative repair due the critical nature of his wound given that the patient is unstable.

Given that the patient is unstable, vascular repair takes precedence over orthopedic repair. While the patient does not demonstrate gross signs of orthopedic injury at this time, the team should x-ray the right femur once the patient is stabilized.

Pro-Tips

- A patient with a high-risk penetrating injury will require a Level 1 Trauma Center.
- Perform a primary survey for all trauma patients. Follow the systematic structure for the primary survey by using the ABCDEs: airway, breathing, circulation, disability, and exposure. Utilize adjuncts as clinically warranted such the FAST exam, chest x-ray, and pelvic x-ray.
- After the primary survey, be sure to perform a secondary to obtain additional history and complete a thorough physical exam to assess for additional injuries.
- Patients who are unstable with a positive finding on the primary or secondary survey should go to the operating room. Patients who are stable can proceed to imaging.
- In patients that sustain penetrating extremity trauma, it is important to assess for hard signs of vascular injury and control active bleeding. Patients that are unstable should undergo operative management immediately. In stable patients, use additional testing modalities such as ABIs or CTA to further assess for signs of vascular injury.
- For patients with signs of orthopedic injury, closed fractures should be externally reduced and internally reduced, before addressing vascular injuries. However, in open fractures, address vascular injuries in the extremity first. It is important to recognize and quickly address compartment syndrome in the acute setting.
- All unstable penetrating trauma patients who demonstrate worsening hemodynamic stability or acute changes in their exam warrant immediate operative management. An

emergency thoracotomy should be performed for patients that have witnessed traumatic arrests less than 15 minutes of pre-hospital CPR following penetrating injury to the torso, less than 5 minutes of prehospital CPR in patients following penetrating injury to the neck or extremity, and patients in profound refractory shock.

References

1. Modrall JG, Weaver FA, Yellin AE. Diagnosis and management of penetrating vascular trauma and the injured extremity. *Emerg Med Clin North Am.* 1998;16 (1):129–144.

2. Newton EJ, Love J. Acute complications of extremity trauma. *Emerg Med Clin North Am.* 2007;25(3):751–761, iv.

3. Southern AP, Celik DH. EMS, Trauma Center Designation. *StatPearls* 2021; www .ncbi.nlm.nih.gov/books/NBK560553/.

4. Marsac ML, Kassam-Adams N, Hildenbrand AK, Nicholls E, Winston FK, Leff SS, Fein J. Implementing a trauma-informed approach in pediatric health care networks. *JAMA Pediatr.* 2016;170(1):70–77.

5. Harris T, Davenport R, Mak M, Brohi K. The evolving science of trauma resuscitation. *Emerg Med Clin North Am.* 2018;36(1):85–106.

6. Quinn AC, Sinert R. What is the utility of the Focused Assessment with Sonography in Trauma (FAST) exam in penetrating torso trauma? *Injury.* 2011;42(5):482–487.

7. Radiology Key: Imaging Chest Trauma. https://radiologykey.com/imaging-chest-trauma/.

8. Hilty MP, Behrendt I, Benneker LM, Martinolli L, Stoupis C, Buggy DJ, Zimmermann H, Exadaktylos AK. Pelvic radiography in ATLS algorithms: a diminishing role? *World J Emerg Surg.* 2008;3:11.

9. Zemaitis MRJ, Planas JH, Waseem M. Trauma secondary survey. *StatPearls* 2021; www.ncbi.nlm.nih.gov/books/NBK441902/.

10. Huber GH, Manna B. Vascular extremity trauma. *StatPearls.* Treasure Island (FL), 2022.

11. Chiu WC, Shanmuganathan K, Mirvis SE, Scalea TM. Determining the need for laparotomy in penetrating torso trauma: a prospective study using triple-contrast enhanced abdominopelvic computed tomography. *J Trauma.* 2001;51 (5):860–868; discussion 868–869.

12. Alao T, Waseem M. Neck trauma. *StatPearls* 2021; www.ncbi.nlm.nih.gov/books/NBK470422/.

13. Shiroff AM, Gale SC, Martin ND, Marchalik D, Petrov D, Ahmed HM, Rotondo MF, Gracias VH. Penetrating neck trauma: a review of management strategies and discussion of the "No Zone" approach. *Am Surg.* 2013;79(1):23–29.

14. Ibraheem K, Khan M, Rhee P, Azim A, O'Keeffe T, Tang A, Kulvatunyou N, Joseph B. "No zone" approach in penetrating neck trauma reduces unnecessary computed tomography angiography and negative explorations. *J Surg Res.* 2018;221:113–120.

15. Nowicki JL, Stew B, Ooi E. Penetrating neck injuries: a guide to evaluation and management. *Ann R Coll Surg Engl.* 2018;100(1):6–11.

16. Tessler RA, Nguyen H, Newton C, Betts J. Pediatric penetrating neck trauma: hard signs of injury and selective neck exploration. *J Trauma Acute Care Surg.* 2017;82(6):989–994.

17. Ball CG. Penetrating nontorso trauma: the extremities. *Can J Surg.* 2015;58(4):286–288.

18. Ivatury RR, Anand R, Ordonez C. Penetrating extremity trauma. *World J Surg.* 2015;39(6):1389–1396.

19. Benabbas R, deSouza IS. Ankle–brachial index for diagnosis of arterial injury in penetrating extremity trauma. *Acad Emerg Med.* 2021;28(8):925–926.

20. Smith AA, Ochoa JE, Wong S, Beatty S, Elder J, Guidry C, McGrew P, McGuinness C, Duchesne J, Schroll R. Prehospital tourniquet use in penetrating extremity trauma: decreased blood transfusions and limb complications. *J Trauma Acute Care Surg.* 2019;86 (1):43–51.

21. le Roux A, Du Plessis AM, Pitcher R. Yield of CT angiography in penetrating lower extremity trauma. *Emerg Radiol.* 2021;28 (4):743–749.

22. Romagnoli AN, DuBose J, Dua A, Betzold R, Bee T, Fabian T, Morrison J, Skarupa D, Podbielski J, Inaba K, Feliciano D, Kauvar D ; AAST PROOVIT Study Group. Hard signs gone soft: A critical evaluation of presenting signs of extremity vascular injury. *J Trauma Acute Care Surg.* 2021;90(1):1–10.

23. Smith JE, Rickard A, Wise D. Traumatic cardiac arrest. *J R Soc Med.* 2015;108 (1):11–16.

24. Teeter W, Haase D. Updates in traumatic cardiac arrest. *Emerg Med Clin North Am.* 2020;38(4):891–901.

25. Ariss AB, Bachir R, El Sayed M. Factors associated with survival in adult patients with traumatic arrest: a retrospective cohort study from US trauma centers. *BMC Emerg Med.* 2021;21(1):77.

26. Avarello JT, Cantor RM. Pediatric major trauma: an approach to evaluation and management. *Emerg Med Clin North Am.* 2007;25(3):803–836, x.

Further Reading

1. The Center for Disease Control and Prevention. 10 Leading Causes of Violence-Related Injury Death, United States. 2020; https://wisqars.cdc.gov/data/lcd/home?lcd=eyJjYXVzZXMiOlsiVklPIl0sInN0YXRlcyI6WyIwMSIsIjAyIiwiMDQiLCIwNSIsIjA2IiwiMDgiLCIwOSIsIjEwIiwiMTEiLCIxMiIsIjEzIiwiMTUiLCIxNiIsIjE3IiwiMTgiLCIxOSIsIjIwIiwiMjEiLCIyMiIsIjIzIiwiMjQiLCIyNSIsIjI2IiwiMjciLCIyOCIsIjI5IiwiMzAiLCIzMSIsIjMyIiwiMzMiLCIzNCIsIjM1IiwiMzYiLCIzNyIsIjM4IiwiMzkiLCI0MCIsIjQxIiwiNDIiLCI0MyIsIjQ0IiwiNDUiLCI0NiIsIjQ3IiwiNDgiLCI0OSIsIjUwIiwiNTEiLCI1MiIsIjUzIiwiNTQiLCI1NSIsIjU2IXSwicmFjZSI6WyIxIiwiMiIsIjMiLCI0Il0sImV0aG5pY2l0eSI6WyIxIiwiMiIsIjMiXSwic2V4IjpbIjEiLCIyIl0sImZyb21ZZWFyIjpbIjAyIXSwidG9ZZWFyIjpbIjAyIXSwibnVtYmVyX29mX3NhdXNlc

yI6WyIxMCJdLCJhZ2VfZ3JvdXBfZm9ybWF0dGluZyI6WyJsY2QxWdlIl0sImN1c3RvbUFnZXNNaW4iOlsiMCJdLCJjdXN0b21BZ2VzTWF4IjpbIjE5OSJdLCJ5cGxseWdlcyI6WyI2NSJdfQ%3D%3D.

2. The Educational Fund to Stop Gun Violence. United States Gun Deaths 2020. https://efsgv.org/state/united-states/.

3. Pino EC, Gebo E, Dugan E, Jay J. Trends in violent penetrating injuries during the first year of the COVID-19 pandemic. *JAMA Netw Open.* 2022;5(2):e2145708.

4. Formica MK. An eye on disparities, health equity, and racism – the case of firearm injuries in urban youth in the United States and globally. *Pediatr Clin North Am.* 2021;68 (2):389–399.

Substance Use

David A. Leon, Arvin K. Jundoria, and Andrew Stolbach

Vignette

A 25-year-old man arrives at the emergency department (ED) in police custody. According to the police officer, the patient was a "drug dealer" and he swallowed packages of drugs prior to arrest. Law enforcement officers ask you to search the patient and turn the material over to them. The patient is asymptomatic. When the patient's history is taken in the presence of police, he denies swallowing anything.

- How should the clinician approach the undifferentiated substance overdose?
- What concerns exist for patients who have "body stuffed" or ingested unknown substances?
- What medical–legal considerations are relevant to this patient's care?

Introduction

It has been estimated that 11% of United States (US) ED patients have substance use disorder.[1] One urban emergency department estimated that nearly 7% of visits were due to illicit drug use.[2] In a large statewide review of ED visits, alcohol use disorder was more prevalent in rural settings while opioid use disorder was more prevalent in urban settings.[3] Substance use leads to harmful outcomes such as acute injuries, overdose, and medical complications. Forensic laboratory data offer some insight on which drugs are commonly used in US cities. (Ethanol is not included in these reports, but is used ubiquitously and considered to be the most commonly used intoxicating drug.) Opioids, sympathomimetics, cannabinoids, and sedatives classes predominate in all US cities (Table 4.1), although there is some regional variation of the specific drugs used among cities. In Baltimore, for example, the top four drugs identified are cocaine, fentanyl, heroin, and tramadol; in Phoenix, the top four are cannabis, fentanyl, heroin, and methamphetamines.

Table 4.1 Common Drugs Identified in Urban Settings by US Forensic Laboratories[4]

Opioids	Sympathomimetics	Cannabinoids	Sedatives
Buprenorphine	Cocaine	Cannabis/THC	Alprazolam
Fentanyl	Eutylone	Cannabidiol	
Heroin	MDMA	Cannabinol	
Tramadol	Methamphetamine		

The coronavirus disease 2019 (COVID-19) pandemic has resulted in an increase in substance use and an increase in ED visits for substance use, especially opioids.[5] The causes are multifactorial, and are likely due to increased isolation and decreased access to care.

Along with the acute problems associated with drug use, the illicit nature begets additional challenges; the urban emergency physician should be able to address the legal and medical issues that are associated with drug use. As the illicit drug supply is not regulated, patients may present with complications of drug adulterants or medical issues from drug smuggling and internal concealment – "body packing" and "body stuffing." There are also legal issues that arise when patients who need medical care are in police custody.

The Acutely Poisoned Patient

Initial management of any poisoned patient includes attention to airway, breathing, circulation, and bedside measurement of glucose. Treatment of a suspected poisoned patient should be guided by the presence of a clinical toxidrome, or the group of signs and symptoms associated with a particular drug. The toxidrome is identified from vital signs and the physical examination, with focus on mental status (sedated or excited), pupil size (pinpoint or dilated), bowel sounds (decreased or increased), and skin (dry or diaphoretic). Because acetaminophen overdose is common and treatable when found early, acetaminophen concentration should be checked in patients with ingestions with the intent of self-harm.[6] Women of childbearing age for pregnancy should be tested for pregnancy.

In the ED, toxidromes can be subdivided into two broad categories: those that cause illness from excessive sedation (such as opioids, sedative-hypnotics) and those that cause illness from agitation (such as sedative-hypnotic withdrawal, opioid withdrawal, or sympathomimetic poisoning).

The Sedated Toxicology Patient

Overview

Sedated ED patients should be promptly evaluated for emergency medical conditions. The differential diagnosis of agitation is broad and includes metabolic, endocrine, neurologic, infectious, traumatic, and psychiatric conditions. Patients can present with one or more of these conditions simultaneously. In this section, we will address common toxicologic causes of sedation. The most common toxicologic causes of sedation include toxicity from opioids or sedative-hypnotics. The overriding principle of management of the sedated toxicology patient is management of respiratory depression.

Opioid Toxicity

The term "opioids" encompasses both synthetic and natural chemicals that bind opioid receptors, while "opiates" refer to those derived from the poppy, *Papaver somniferum*. We avoid the term "narcotic" because it refers to opioids in a medical context but describes any illicit drug when used in a legal context.

Activation of opioid receptors in the brain and spinal cord results in analgesia, euphoria, and respiratory depression in a dose-dependent manner. In addition to ingestion and insufflation (snorting), opioids can be administered by intravenous or subcutaneous ("skin popping") routes. Common opioids used in the urban setting are the full agonists fentanyl (and its analogs), heroin, and prescription opioids. Opioid deaths are a result of hypercapnia and hypoxia from respiratory depression (Table 4.2).

Opioid Toxicity Management

The key to the management of opioid poisoning is the restoration of ventilation. As soon as hypoventilation is recognized, ventilate the patient by bag-valve mask. Administer naloxone, a short-acting competitive opioid antagonist, for respiratory depression. The goal of naloxone administration is to restore ventilation, not to diagnose opioid poisoning or normalize mental status.

There is no "one-size-fits-all" naloxone dose. The ideal naloxone dose is sufficient to restore ventilation without precipitating withdrawal. In the adult, we recommend an initial dose of 0.04 mg by intravenous route. The dose is increased in 2-minute increments if the first dose does not produce a response.[7]

The most commonly recommended naloxone dosing progression (mg) is 0.04, 0.4, 2, 4, 10.[8]

If intravenous access is not readily available, naloxone should be administered by intranasal or subcutaneous route, although these routes may require more naloxone and are harder to titrate because of slower absorption. If a patient has received 10–20 mg of naloxone without improvement of ventilation, reconsider the diagnosis. In these patients, further naloxone is unlikely to be effective and you should consider securing the airway by other means (e.g., intubation).

There are many caveats to the above guidance. Patients with ingestions of methadone or other long-acting oral opioids should be observed for longer periods. If the patient ingested a large amount of opioids, there may be late absorption of drug, leading to clinical manifestations occurring hours after naloxone reversal. Consider a longer period of monitoring for patients who have received large doses (2–4 mg) of naloxone (due to delayed naloxone absorption).

If there is a question of whether the patient intended to overdose to harm themself, the patient should have a risk assessment for suicidality. All patients with opioid use disorder should be referred for substance use treatment. If possible, patients should be given follow-up appointments while still in the ED. Emergency department-based peer-support programs may be ideal in this role.[9] Patients discharged after opioid overdose should be provided with naloxone and those who inject should be counseled on safe injection practices.

Sedative-Hypnotic Toxicity

Ethanol (common alcohol), benzodiazepines, barbiturates, and other common drugs collectively cause the sedative-hypnotic toxidrome. Globally, 5.9% of deaths are attributed to

Table 4.2 Clinical Features of Patients with Opioid Toxidrome

Vital signs	**Blood pressure:** Decreased
	Heart rate: Decreased
	Respiratory rate: Decreased
Mental status	Sedation, coma
Physical examination	**Eyes:** Constricted pupils
	GI: Decreased bowel sounds
	Skin: Cool skin

ethanol.[10] Ethanol activates inhibitory gamma-aminobutyric acid (GABA) receptors and inhibits excitatory glutamate receptors.[11] Benzodiazepines and barbiturates result in increased GABA tone. In most cases, these substances cause sedation and upper airway relaxation but not true respiratory depression. (In large ethanol ingestions or combined sedative-hypnotic and opioid toxicity, respiratory depression may be present; Table 4.3.)

Sedative-Hypnotic Toxicity Management

The key to sedative-hypnotic toxicity management is support of breathing and exclusion of other medical and traumatic illnesses. Patients may have obstruction from upper airway relaxation as opposed to true respiratory depression. In most cases, patient positioning is sufficient for opening the airway. Use an oral airway when needed to maintain upper airway patency. If patient positioning does not help, intubation may be necessary. Monitor with pulse oximetry and capnometry to identify hypoventilation. Perform a physical examination to identify traumatic injury. If head injury cannot be excluded by history and examination, obtain computed tomography (CT) imaging. In patients with mild alcohol intoxication and clear history, diagnostic testing is unnecessary.

Administer naloxone if opioid co-ingestion is suspected. Other reversal agents, such as flumazenil, are rarely helpful. Flumazenil is a competitive benzodiazepine antagonist. Although it can reverse hypoventilation from benzodiazepines, it may cause seizures in patients with benzodiazepine tolerance, and strong consideration should be given to consulting with a toxicologist before using it.[12,13]

Serum ethanol level rarely contributes to management in alcohol intoxication. A serum alcohol concentration of 150 mg/dL, for example, may be consistent with intoxication in an inexperienced drinker, but withdrawal in a frequent drinker. If an ethanol level is obtained, a "high" serum ethanol concentration does not rule out comorbid conditions, but a "low" ethanol concentration in a sedated patient is an indicator to escalate the diagnostic evaluation.

Patients are safe for discharge when they are clinically "sober." Sobriety (absence of intoxication) is a clinical diagnosis. The duration of observation needed for sobriety depends on the specific substance and the amount ingested. Discharge should not be based on an ethanol level. Patients are safe for discharge when they have a stable gait and reasonable judgment. The decision to hold a patient against their will is ethically and legally fraught, and there is no single strategy for balancing patient autonomy with the clinician's duty to protect the patient and others from harm. Clinical judgment must prevail.

Table 4.3 Clinical Features of Patients with Sedative-Hypnotic Toxidrome

Vital signs	**Blood pressure:** Normal or decreased **Heart rate:** Normal or decreased **Respiratory rate:** Decreased **Temperature:** Decreased
Mental status	Disinhibition, sedation, coma
Physical examination	**Neuro:** Unsteady gait, uncoordinated, slurred speech,

Agitated Patient

Overview

Patients who present to the ED in an agitated state must be quickly and safely stabilized to allow for the prompt recognition and management of emergency medical conditions.

The differential diagnosis of agitation is broad and includes metabolic, endocrine, neurologic, infectious, and psychiatric conditions. Patients can present with one or more of these conditions simultaneously. This section will address common toxicologic causes of agitation. The chapter on "Disruptive and Dangerous Agitation" provides details on management.

Sympathomimetic Toxicity

Sympathomimetics are stimulants that activate the sympathetic nervous system. The sympathomimetic toxidrome is caused by increased concentration of biogenic amines (norepinephrine, dopamine, serotonin) at the preganglionic synapse, resulting in increased sympathetic tone. Common sympathomimetics in the urban setting include methamphetamine, MDMA, methylphenidate cocaine, and synthetic cathinones ("bath salts" such as mephedrone).[14] Sympathomimetics can be injected, insufflated, ingested, or absorbed across mucous membranes.

Diagnosis of sympathomimetic poisoning is based on clinical manifestations and history. It is not possible (or necessary) to identify the specific drug by examination alone. Death from sympathomimetic toxicity is associated with hyperthermia, which is the result of increased heat generation from muscular contraction and decreased heat dissipation from vasoconstriction. Mortality from cocaine overdose, for instance, is 33% higher when ambient temperature exceeds 88°F/31°C[15] (Table 4.4).

Cannabis and Synthetic Cannabinoid Toxicity

The main psychoactive component of the cannabis plant is delta-9-tetrahydrocannabinol (THC). Although tetrahydrocannabinols are still classified as Schedule 1 controlled substances by the United States Drug Enforcement Administration (DEA), cannabis is legal or available for medical use in many states. Synthetic cannabinoids, first reported in the US in 2008, are analogs of THC. There are hundreds of known synthetic cannabinoids. Originally

Table 4.4 Clinical Features of Patients with Sympathomimetic Toxidrome

Vital signs	**Blood pressure:** Increased **Heart rate:** Increased **Respiratory rate:** Increased **Body temperature:** Increased
Mental status	Agitated, disoriented, combative
Physical examination	**Neuro:** Tremors and seizure-like activity **Eyes:** Mydriasis, rapid eye movements **Abdomen:** Decreased bowel sounds and slowed digestion **Skin:** Warm, flushed, diaphoretic

used as research chemicals, many are marketed as "incense" or "herbal" products under various names including: "K2," "spice," and many others.[16] Despite initially being sold commercially in many urban areas, most are ultimately classified as Schedule 1 controlled substances as soon as they are identified by the United States Drug Enforcement Administration.

Activation of brain CB1 receptors is responsible for many of the consequential clinical manifestations of cannabinoids. The effects of THC are generally mild at typical doses. Most users experience mild effects and do not seek medical care. However, high doses of THC or synthetic cannabinoids that cause excessive CB1 receptor activation result in toxic or even life-threatening effects (Table 4.5).

Management of Acute Agitation from Sympathomimetics or Cannabinoids

As with any patient, initial assessment includes ensuring airway and breathing are secured while assessing circulation. Bedside glucose should be checked in all patients with change in mental status or a neurologic deficit.

The key principle of management of acutely agitated patient is to prevent and treat hyperthermia and metabolic abnormalities. Measure core body temperature to diagnose hyperthermia. Employ rapid external cooling for patients with temperature 39°C or greater. Use ice water immersion or evaporative cooling with the goal of reducing temperature to 39°C within 30 minutes. We do not recommend air-circulating cooling blankets, which cool too slowly. Endovascular cooling may achieve good cooling rates, but the requirement for setup and cannulation makes overall initiation too slow. For severe hyperthermia coupled with agitation, a paralytic may be employed (with mechanical ventilation) to rapidly stop muscular heat production.

Alcohol Withdrawal

Frequent use of any sedative-hypnotic will lead to tolerance – where patients need the substance to maintain normal physiologic function. In tolerant individuals, discontinuation of the sedative-hypnotic results in withdrawal.

Patients can experience withdrawal from any sedative-hypnotic. In practice, ethanol withdrawal is more common than withdrawal from benzodiazepines or barbiturates, although the same management principles apply to treating withdrawal from any drug in those classes.

Table 4.5 Clinical Features of Patients with Cannabinoid Toxicity

Vital signs	**Blood pressure:** Increased **Heart rate:** Increased (although occasionally decreased) **Respiratory rate:** Increased (although respiratory depression can occur at very high doses) **Temperature:** Increased
Mental status	Agitation, somnolence, delirium, inattention
Physical exam	**Neuro:** Seizures, psychosis **Eyes:** Conjunctival injection, nystagmus **Cardiac:** Ventricular tachycardia (occasional sinus bradycardia)

The loss of ethanol inhibition results in central nervous system excitation, manifesting in a spectrum from mild irritability and tremor to tachycardia, hypertension, seizures, and delirium.

History should identify frequency of alcohol use and timing of the patient's last drink. Patients with high intake who recently stopped drinking are likely to experience severe withdrawal. Perhaps most importantly, the patient should be asked why they stopped or slowed their alcohol intake. In many cases, decrease in drinking was caused by an underlying medical condition such as pancreatitis, alcoholic ketoacidosis, or others. Identification and treatment of the underlying condition will ultimately be just as important as treating withdrawal symptoms (Table 4.6).

Alcohol withdrawal presents in a classic spectrum ranging from mild withdrawal to delirium tremens (Table 4.7).

Alcohol Withdrawal Management

Benzodiazepines are established as safe and effective first-line treatment for most patients in alcohol withdrawal. This class of medications treats seizures and irritability while causing minimal respiratory depression. Symptom-triggered dosing is superior to a fixed dosing schedule. We recommend use of a withdrawal severity scale to titrate benzodiazepine dosing. The 10-item Clinical Institute Withdrawal Assessment Alcohol Scale Revised (CIWA-Ar) has

Table 4.6 Clinical Features of Sedative-Hypnotic Withdrawal

Vital signs	**Blood pressure:** Increased **Heart rate:** Increased **Respiratory rate:** Increased **Temperature:** Increased
Mental status	Agitated, delirious
Physical examination	**Neuro:** Seizures, hallucinations, headache, tremors **Cardiac:** Tachycardia **Skin:** Diaphoresis

Table 4.7 Alcohol Withdrawal Syndromes

Alcohol Withdrawal Syndrome	Timing After Last Drink	Key Clinical Features
Uncomplicated withdrawal	>6 h	Tachycardia Tremor Diaphoresis
Alcoholic epilepsy	~24 h	Brief generalized tonic–clonic seizure
Alcoholic hallucinosis	>2 days	Tactile or visual hallucinations with clear sensorium
Delirium tremens	3–4 days (can last for weeks)	Autonomic instability Psychomotor agitation Delirium

been found to be useful, as has the shorter 5-item Brief Alcohol Withdrawal Scale (BAWS; Table 4.8).[16]

Dosing of benzodiazepines should follow a symptom-triggered approach based on CIWA-Ar or BAWS. The choice of specific agent may depend on clinician preference or institutional protocol. Regardless of the benzodiazepine selected, attention should be paid to remaining consistent through the patient's care, as mixing benzodiazepines with varying times of onset, potencies, and durations of action can create unnecessary complexity to the management.

A minority of patients are refractory to high doses of benzodiazepines and may benefit from phenobarbital. We recommend IV phenobarbital administered every 30 minutes up to a maximum dose of 260 mg, holding for respiratory depression. "Up front" phenobarbital – giving phenobarbital before benzodiazepines – may be beneficial in patients with a history of severe alcohol or benzodiazepine-refractory withdrawal. Close attention to monitoring respiratory status is necessary when using Phenobarbital with benzodiazepines.

Finally, in addition to treating withdrawal directly, thiamine should be administered, even to patients who do not have features of Wernicke's encephalopathy (such as confusion, ataxia, or ophthalmoplegia). A dose of 100–200 mg IM or IV is appropriate, with higher dosing indicated for patients presenting with seizure or delirium.[17]

Table 4.8 The Brief Alcohol Withdrawal Scale (BAWS)

Tremor	Diaphoresis/sweats
0 No tremor	0 No tremor
1 Not visible, but can be felt	1 Mild, barely visible
2 Moderate with arms extended	2 Beads of sweat
3 At rest, without arms extended	3 Drenching sweats
RAAS (Evaluate level of agitation using the Richmond Agitation–Sedation Scale)	**Confusion/orientation** (Disorientation to time, e.g., by more than 2 days or wrong month or wrong year; disorientation to place, e.g., name of building, city, state)
0 Alert and calm	0 Oriented to person, place, time
1 Restless, anxious, apprehensive, movements not aggressive	1 Disoriented to time or to place but not both
2 Agitated, frequent non-purposeful movement	2 Disoriented to time and placed
3/4 Very agitated, combative, violent	3 Disoriented to person
Hallucinations (Visual, auditory, tactile)	**Total score:** ____ (The total score is the sum of all 5 items)
0 None	Score: 0–1 Mild
1 Vague report, reality testing intact	2–5 Moderate
2 More defined hallucinations	6–15 Severe
3 Obviously responding to internal stimuli, poor reality testing	

Opioid Withdrawal

Opioid withdrawal results from cessation of regular opioid use, and patients present with a spectrum of severity ranging from mild discomfort and flu-like symptoms to severe abdominal pain and irritability (Table 4.9). Iatrogenic withdrawal, from antagonist administration, is particularly severe and can be marked by life-threatening catecholamine release.

Opioid Withdrawal Management

Severity of opioid withdrawal can be quantified with the Clinical Opiate Withdrawal Scale (COWS; Table 4.10).[18]

For treatment, opioid agonist therapy is preferable for most patients. Medications for opioid use disorder (MOUD) such as buprenorphine, methadone, or naltrexone are considered to be superior to abstinence-based programs. There are apparent advantages to initiating therapy in the ED. Initiation of buprenorphine in the ED was found to increase engagement in addiction treatment and reduce illicit opioid use at 30 days when compared to referral alone.[19] In a retrospective review, ED buprenorphine prescriptions were associated with decreased hospitalizations and decreased overdoses at 1 year.[20]

Methadone is a full mu-opioid agonist that binds to the mu receptors and can alleviate symptoms for 24 hours or longer.[21] Buprenorphine is a partial mu-opioid agonist with high affinity for opioid receptors. As a partial agonist, buprenorphine is less likely to cause significant respiratory depression. Buprenorphine can precipitate withdrawal in opioid intoxicated patients, but this can be alleviated by administering more buprenorphine.[22]

Non-opioid medications are preferable in patients who have received antagonists, and in whom agonists are therefore unlikely to work. Clonidine, benzodiazepines, antiemetics, and/or antispasmodics may be given for symptomatic relief.

Urine Drug Screen

Emergency department urine toxicology testing is common even though the clinical utility is limited. Urine drug tests in the hospital setting are typically immunoassays, which are rapid, relatively inexpensive, and easy to automate. This contrasts with chromatographic tests, which are considered "gold standard" and used in legal settings.

There are several limitations of urine immunoassays. Immunoassays use antibodies, and substances with similar structure to the target can cause false positives. For example,

Table 4.9 Clinical Features of Opioid Withdrawal

Vital signs	**Blood pressure:** Increased
	Heart rate: Increased
	Respiratory rate: Increased
	Temperature: Normal
Mental status	Normal mental status
Physical examination	**Constitutional:** Restless
	Eyes: Dilated pupils (mydriasis)
	Nose: Rhinorrhea
	Mouth: Yawning
	GI: Increased bowel sounds, nausea, vomiting, diarrhea
	Skin: Diaphoresis, piloerection

Table 4.10 Clinical Opiate Withdrawal Scale (COWS)

Resting pulse rate:____beats/minute
(Measured after the patient is sitting or lying for 1 minute)
0 Pulse rate 80 or below
1 Pulse rate 81–100
2 Pulse rate 101–120
4 Pulse rate >120

GI upset: *(over last 1/2 hour)*
0 No GI symptoms
1 Stomach cramps
2 Nausea or loose stool
3 Vomiting or diarrhea
5 Multiple episodes of diarrhea or vomiting

Sweating: *(over past 1/2 hour, not accounted for by room temperature or patient activity)*
0 No report of chills or flushing
1 Subjective report of chills or flushing
2 Flushed or observable moistness on face
3 Beads of sweat on brow or face
4 Sweat streaming off face

Tremor: *(observation of outstretched hands)*
0 No tremor
1 Tremor can be felt, but not observed
3 Slight tremor observable
4 Gross tremor or muscle twitching

Restlessness: *(Observation during assessment)*
0 Able to sit still
1 Reports difficulty sitting still, but is able to do so
3 Frequent shifting or extraneous movements of legs/arms
5 Unable to sit still for more than a few seconds

Yawning: *(Observation during assessment)*
0 No yawning
1 Yawning once or twice during assessment
2 Yawning three or more times during assessment
4 Yawning several times/minute

Pupil size:
0 Pupils pinned or normal size for room light
1 Pupils possibly larger than normal for room light
2 Pupils moderately dilated
5 Pupils so dilated that only the rim of the iris is visible

Anxiety or irritability:
0 None
1 Patient reports increasing irritability or anxiousness
2 Patient obviously irritable or anxious
4 Patient so irritable or anxious that participation in the assessment is difficult

Bone or joint aches: *(If patient was having pain previously, only additional component attributed to opiates withdrawal is scored)*
0 Not present
1 Mild diffuse discomfort
2 Patient reports severe diffuse aching of joints/muscles
4 Patient is rubbing joints or muscles and is unable to sit still because of discomfort

Gooseflesh skin:
0 Skin is smooth
3 Piloerection of skin can be felt or hairs standing up on arms
5 Prominent piloerection

Runny nose or tearing: *(Not accounted for by cold symptoms or allergies)*
0 Not present
1 Nasal stuffiness or unusually moist eyes
2 Nose running or tearing
4 Nose constantly running or tears streaming down cheeks

Total score:____(The total score is the sum of all 11 items)
Score:
5–12 Mild
13–24 Moderate
25–36 Moderately Severe
>36 Severe

dextromethorphan (found in non-prescription antitussives) can cause false positive phencyclidine (PCP) result.[23]

Furthermore, as urine tests look for drug or metabolite in urine (not in blood or end organs), the detection window is often longer than the duration of effect.

Urine drug immunoassay panels typically look for common drugs, but they are not intended to be comprehensive. Most clinical panels test for common opiates, benzodiazepines, amphetamine, phencyclidine, and cannabis. Some panels also look for fentanyl and will also identify some structurally similar fentanyl analogs. However, hospital panels do not identify synthetic cannabinoids, many benzodiazepines (such as lorazepam or clonazepam), or other emerging drugs.[24]

Drug testing should only be performed to answer a specific clinical question for treatment of the patient, such as screening a pediatric patient for an exposure, or in the case of a new and undifferentiated mania or psychosis. Immunoassays are not used for high-stakes or forensic applications. These assays are not specific as chromatographic tests and clinical settings do not maintain chain of custody.

Drug testing should never be performed only at the request of legal authorities. If a law enforcement officer desires a specimen, they will have a procedure for obtaining the specimen on their own. Hospital legal assistance should be contacted in real time if law enforcement requests specimen collection by clinical staff.

Adulterants

By nature, the illicit drug supply is not regulated for purity or quality control. Illicit drugs commonly contain additional pharmacologically active components added to increase the bulk of the product or enhance the potency of the primary active components, and these adulterants or "cutting agents" can be harmful. Adulterants are typically underreported in the clinical setting, and vary significantly by geographic region.

Brodifacoum

For reasons that are unclear, the long-acting vitamin K-antagonist (or "superwarfarin") brodifacoum has been found in synthetic cannabinoids. Typically used as a rodenticide, brodifacoum does not have known psychoactive effects. It is not known if the presence of brodifacoum in some synthetic cannabinoids is intentional or malicious. The diagnosis should be suspected in patients with a history of synthetic cannabinoid use presenting with unexplained bruising, hematuria, or bleeding. An elevated INR is suggestive, but specialized testing for brodifacoum is required to confirm the diagnosis. Patients have required long-term oral vitamin K therapy.[25]

Diphenhydramine

This non-prescription antihistamine with sedative and anticholinergic properties has been found as adulterant in illicit drugs including cocaine, heroin, and methamphetamine.[26] Diphenhydramine elicits central nervous system (CNS) effects, including euphoria, agitation, hallucinations, and delirium. Its rapid entrance into the CNS causes significant sedation, as well as anticholinergic effects (such as blurred vision, dry mouth, urinary retention, impotence, tachycardia), and gastrointestinal effects (such as nausea and constipation). In overdoses, severe effects from diphenhydramine can include tachycardia, *torsades de pointes*, delirium, and seizures.[27]

Levamisole

Levamisole is a veterinary and human antihelminthic drug commonly found as an adulterant in cocaine. It is estimated by the US DEA to be present in nearly 80% of cocaine seized in the United States.[28] Levamisole may potentiate cocaine's psychostimulant effects. It has been linked to debilitating, and sometimes fatal, immunologic effects in cocaine users, including vasculitis, agranulocytosis, leukopenia, purpura, and necrotized skin tissue.[29]

Talc

Talc is a mineral used for anti-stick or anti-cake properties in cosmetics and other products, and can be used as filler by sellers, to "cut" or increase the ratio of volume to actual drug. When injected, talc can cause granulomatosis, pulmonary hypertension, and pulmonary infarction.[30]

Xylazine

Xylazine is an imidazoline (like clonidine or oxymetazoline) used in veterinary medicine as a sedative with muscle relaxant and analgesic properties. In humans, xylazine acts as a CNS depressant resulting in respiratory depression, bradycardia, and hypotension. Increasingly found in the US illicit fentanyl and heroin supply, xylazine, and can potentiate opioid sedation and respiratory depression. Because xylazine is not an opioid, it does not respond to opioid reversal agents such as naloxone; therefore, if illicit opioid products containing xylazine are used, naloxone might be less effective in fully reversing an overdose. Several states have reported increases in xylazine-involved overdose deaths, in particular in the Northeast US.[31]

Law Enforcement and Legal Issues Related to ED Patients and Substance Use

Law enforcement officers (LEO) may be present in the ED in a variety of roles: Providing facility security, guarding patients in their custody, collecting evidence, documenting injuries, and investigating reports of abuse. Because of the illicit status of many drugs, patients with substance use may be in the custody of LEO.

The presence of LEO should not adversely affect the delivery of patient care.[32] In the ED, the presence of LEO may diminish patient trust in clinicians, especially in patients in custody or under police investigation. Patients may not be willing to disclose important health information (such as drug use) in the presence of LEO. When possible, clinicians should collect history outside the presence of LEO. When officers must be present, the clinician should recognize that the presence of law enforcement may affect the ability to obtain an accurate history.

It is the duty of the clinician to maintain patient welfare as their primary responsibility. Patients should receive equal respect and attention regardless of their status as prisoners or subjects of law enforcement investigation. Patients in police custody maintain the same rights to accept or refuse medical care as other patients.

Clinician Reporting Information to Law Enforcement

The patient–physician relationship is built on the assumption of respect for patient privacy and protection of confidentiality. Clinicians may only disclose information to LEO under specific conditions, and should be familiar with how patient privacy and confidentiality relate to mandatory reporting regulations.

Test results (including drug testing) should not be disclosed to LEO, nor should tests be performed at their behest. Health Insurance Portability and Accountability Act (HIPAA) regulations and state laws offer guidance regarding protected health information (PHI) information that should be reported to authorities. There are some situations (such as statute or a court order; when confidentiality threatens to cause harm to others; cases of gunshot or knife wounds; or for the collection, preservation, and sharing of physical evidence and medical information in regard to possible criminal acts) in which information sharing with LEO may be permissible, and clinicians should contact their institutional legal department in real time when uncertainty arises.[33]

Body "Stuffing" and "Packing" of Drugs

Patients may present to the ED following internal concealment or ingestion of illicit substances. "Body stuffing" is unplanned and hasty ingestion of material, usually to evade law enforcement. "Body packing" is a preplanned ingestion of a large amount of drug for the purpose of smuggling.

Body Stuffing

"Stuffing" typically involves internal concealment of smaller quantities of drug which are poorly packaged for ingestion, if packaged at all. The intent is usually to rapidly hide or dispose of a substance. Patients usually ingest the material, although it may be hidden in the rectum or vagina. Because these drugs are loosely packed, the drug is likely to leak out and be absorbed into systemic circulation.

For oral ingestion, patients should be offered activated charcoal if they are not at risk of aspiration. Rectal and vaginal packets should be removed with patient consent. Symptomatic patients should be treated based on the prevailing toxidrome, and asymptomatic patients should be observed for at least 6 hours, to identify symptoms of delayed drug absorption.[34]

Body Packing

"Packing" is the intentional ingestion of well-packaged drugs (usually opioids or cocaine) for the purpose of smuggling, and the smuggler intends to recover the packets intact once safely beyond the scrutiny of authorities. Body packer drug packet construction is sophisticated, so packets are unlikely to leak. However, because of the large quantity of drugs ingested, any packet rupture that occurs could be clinically catastrophic to the packer. Patients may present for medical care if taken into custody (often at an airport) or if they are symptomatic from package rupture or obstruction.

Radiographic evaluation should be performed on suspected body packers, and non-contrast CT has a higher sensitivity for identifying packets and obstruction than plain radiographs.[35] Establish intravenous access and cardiac monitoring. Perform whole bowel irrigation by administering polyethylene glycol electrolyte lavage solution until all packets have passed. Surgical removal should be performed for rupture of cocaine packets or mechanical obstruction of any type of packet.

Patients require admission for monitoring until all packets are passed or removed.[36]

For symptomatic patients with concern for small bowel obstruction or symptomatic patients with symptoms consistent with sympathomimetic toxidrome, obtain emergent surgical consultation.

Vignette Conclusion

The patient is initially awake and alert and has a stable airway, breathing, and circulation. Even though police remain by his side, you let him know that you are here to help him and make sure he receives good medical care. You inform him that he has the right to accept or refuse any treatment. He declines to say what he swallowed, but law enforcement thinks he was carrying heroin. You offer activated charcoal, but he declines. The law enforcement officer asks if you can perform a drug test, but you inform them that you will only perform tests for medical necessity and that you cannot disclose test results to them.

An hour after initial evaluation, the patient becomes sleepy. His pupils are small, bowel sounds decreased, and respiration is slow. You diagnose an opioid toxidrome and administer 0.4 mg of IV naloxone. His breathing normalizes and you monitor him with pulse oximetry. His breathing remains normal for 6 hours of observation. You ask him if he would like to speak to a peer recovery specialty about opioid use disorder treatment options, but he says that he does not usually use drugs. He declines any other medical concerns and you discharge him into police custody.

Pro-Tips

- Common drug classes in urban areas include opioids, sympathomimetics, cannabinoids, alcohol, and other sedatives.
- In the acutely poisoned patient, address airway, breathing, and circulation, check blood glucose, and then administer further treatment based on the presence of a toxidrome.
- Sedated toxicology patients (sedative-hypnotic and opioid toxidromes) require support of airway and ventilation.
- When giving naloxone, "start low and go slow." The goal of treatment is to restart breathing and avoid withdrawal, not to wake patients up.
- Hyperthermia kills sympathomimetic poisoned patients. These patients need management of psychomotor agitation and rapid management of hyperthermia.
- In patients with alcohol withdrawal, find out why they stopped drinking. Did they stop because they were feeling sick? Identification and treatment of an underlying condition will ultimately be just as important as treating withdrawal.
- For patients in alcohol withdrawal who have been admitted to the intensive care unit for refractory alcohol withdrawal, it may be useful to initiate phenobarbital up front.
- Urine drug screens rarely contribute to acute management. These tests are not specific, not comprehensive, and remain positive for a longer period of time than drug effects last.
- Patients in custody of law enforcement officers have the same right to refuse medical care as any other patient.
- Except in specific situations specified by HIPAA and local laws, confidential patient health information should not be shared with law enforcement officers.

References

1. Zhang X, Wang N, Hou F, Ali Y, Dora-Laskey A, Dahlem CH, McCabe SE. Emergency department visits by patients with substance use disorder in the United States. *West J Emerg Med.* 2021;22(5):1076–1085. doi: 10.5811/ westjem.2021.3.50839. PMID: 34546883; PMCID: PMC8463055.

2. Binks S, Hoskins R, Salmon D, Benger J. Prevalence and healthcare burden of illegal drug use among emergency department

patients. *Emerg Med J.* 2005;22 (12):872–873. doi: 10.1136/ emj.2004.022665. PMID: 16299197; PMCID: PMC1726620.

3. Xierali IM, Day PG, Kleinschmidt KC, Strenth C, Schneider FD, Kale NJ. Emergency department presentation of opioid use disorder and alcohol use disorder. *J Subst Abuse Treat.* 2021;127:108343. doi: 10.1016/j.jsat.2021.108343. Epub 2021 Mar 3. PMID: 34134862

4. www.nflis.deadiversion.usdoj.gov/nflisdata/ docs/NFLISDrug2020AnnualReport.pdf

5. Venkatesh AK, Janke AT, Kinsman J, Rothenberg C, Goyal P, Malicki C, D'Onofrio G, Taylor A, Hawk K. Emergency department utilization for substance use disorders and mental health conditions during COVID-19. *PLoS One.* 2022;17(1):e0262136. doi: 10.1371/journal. pone.0262136. PMID: 35025921; PMCID: PMC8757912.

6. Ashbourne JF, Olson KR, Khayam-Bashi H. Value of rapid screening for acetaminophen in all patients with intentional drug overdose. *Ann Emerg Med.* 1989;18(10):1035–1038. doi:10.1016/ s0196-0644(89)80925-4. PMID: 2802276.

7. Boyer EW. Management of opioid analgesic overdose. *N Engl J Med.* 2012;367(2):146–155. doi: 10.1056/ NEJMra1202561. PMID: 22784117; PMCID: PMC3739053.

8. Connors NJ, Nelson LS. The evolution of recommended naloxone dosing for opioid overdose by medical specialty. *J Med Toxicol.* 2016;12(3):276–281. doi: 10.1007/s13181-016-0559-3. Epub 2016 Jun 7. PMID: 27271032; PMCID: PMC4996792.

9. McGuire AB, Powell KG, Treitler PC, Wagner KD, Smith KP, Cooperman N, Robinson L, Carter J, Ray B, Watson DP. Emergency department-based peer support for opioid use disorder: emergent functions and forms. *J Subst Abuse Treat.* 2020;108:82–87. doi: 10.1016/j. jsat.2019.06.013. Epub 2019 Jun 19. PMID: 31280928; PMCID: PMC7393771.

10. World Health Organization. *Global Status Report on Alcohol and Health.* World Health Organization, 2014.

11. Banerjee N. Neurotransmitters in alcoholism: a review of neurobiological and genetic studies. *Indian J Hum Genet.* 2014;20(1):20–31. doi: 10.4103/0971-6866.132750. PMID: 24959010; PMCID: PMC4065474.

12. Weinbroum AA, Flaishon R, Sorkine P, Szold O, Rudick V. A risk-benefit assessment of flumazenil in the management of benzodiazepine overdose. *Drug Saf.* 1997;17(3):181–196. doi: 10.2165/00002018-199717030-00004. PMID: 9306053.

13. Seger DL. Flumazenil – treatment or toxin. *J Toxicol Clin Toxicol.* 2004;42(2):209–216. doi: 10.1081/clt-120030946. PMID: 15214628.

14. Gonin P, Beysard N, Yersin B, Carron PN. Excited delirium: a systematic review. *Acad Emerg Med.* 2018;25(5):552–565. doi: 10.1111/acem.13330. Epub 2017 Nov 27. PMID: 28990246.

15. Marzuk PM, Tardiff K, Leon AC, Hirsch CS, Portera L, Iqbal MI, Nock MK, Hartwell N. Ambient temperature and mortality from unintentional cocaine overdose. *JAMA.* 1998;279(22):1795–1800. doi: 10.1001/ jama.279.22.1795. PMID: 9628710.

16. Trecki J, Gerona RR, Schwartz MD. Synthetic cannabinoid-related illnesses and deaths. *N Engl J Med.* 2015;373(2):103–107. doi: 10.1056/NEJMp1505328. PMID: 26154784.

17. Praharaj SK, Munoli RN, Shenoy S, Udupa ST, Thomas LS. High-dose thiamine strategy in Wernicke–Korsakoff syndrome and related thiamine deficiency conditions associated with alcohol use disorder. *Indian J Psychiatry.* 2021;63 (2):121–126. doi: 10.4103/psychiatry. IndianJPsychiatry_440_20. Epub 2021 Apr 14. PMID: 34194054; PMCID: PMC8214134.

18. Wesson DR, Ling W. The Clinical Opiate Withdrawal Scale (COWS). *J Psychoactive Drugs.* 2003;35(2):253–259. doi: 10.1080/

02791072.2003.10400007. PMID: 12924748.

19. D'Onofrio G, Chawarski MC, O'Connor PG, Pantalon MV, Busch SH, Owens PH, Hawk K, Bernstein SL, Fiellin DA. Emergency department-initiated buprenorphine for opioid dependence with continuation in primary care: outcomes during and after intervention. *J Gen Intern Med.* 2017;32 (6):660–666. doi: 10.1007/s11606-017-3993-2. Epub 2017 Feb 13. PMID: 28194688; PMCID: PMC5442013.

20. Le T, Cordial P, Sankoe M, Purnode C, Parekh A, Baker T, Hiestand B, Peacock WF, Neuenschwander J. Healthcare use after buprenorphine prescription in a community emergency department: a cohort study. *West J Emerg Med.* 2021;22(6):1270–1275. doi: 10.5811/ westjem.2021.6.51306. PMID: 34787550; PMCID: PMC8597690.

21. Su MK, Lopez JH, Crossa A, Hoffman RS. Low dose intramuscular methadone for acute mild to moderate opioid withdrawal syndrome. *Am J Emerg Med.* 2018;36:1951.

22. Oakley B, Wilson H, Hayes V, Lintzeris N. Managing opioid withdrawal precipitated by buprenorphine with buprenorphine. *Drug Alcohol Rev.* 2021;40(4):567–571. doi: 10.1111/dar.13228. Epub 2021 Jan 21. PMID: 33480051; PMCID: PMC8248003.

23. Hughey JJ, Colby JM. Discovering cross-reactivity in urine drug screening immunoassays through large-scale analysis of electronic health records. *Clin Chem.* 2019;65(12):1522–1531. doi: 10.1373/ clinchem.2019.305409. Epub 2019 Oct 2. PMID: 31578215; PMCID: PMC7055671.

24. Mahajan G. Role of urine drug testing in the current opioid epidemic. *Anesth Analg.* 2017;125(6):2094–2104. doi: 10.1213/ ANE.0000000000002565. PMID: 29189366.

25. Kelkar AH, Smith NA, Martial A, Moole H, Tarantino MD, Roberts JC. An outbreak of synthetic cannabinoid-associated coagulopathy in Illinois. *N Engl J Med.* 2018;379(13):1216–1223. doi: 10.1056/ NEJMoa1807652. PMID: 30280655.

26. www.annemergmed.com/article/S0196-06 44(21)00921-5/fulltext

27. Varma A, Ford L, Patel N, Vale JA. Elimination half-life of diphenhydramine in overdose. *Clin Toxicol (Phila).* 2017;55(6):615–616. doi: 10.1080/ 15563650.2017.1296153. Epub 2017 Mar 28. PMID: 28349707.

28. Tallarida CS, Egan E, Alejo GD, Raffa R, Tallarida RJ, Rawls SM. Levamisole and cocaine synergism: a prevalent adulterant enhances cocaine's action *in vivo.* *Neuropharmacology.* 2014;79:590–595. doi: 10.1016/j.neuropharm.2014.01.002. Epub 2014 Jan 15. PMID: 24440755; PMCID: PMC3989204.

29. Midthun KM, Nelson LS, Logan BK. Levamisole – a toxic adulterant in illicit drug preparations: a review. *Ther Drug Monit.* 2021;43(2):221–228. doi: 10.1097/ FTD.0000000000000851. PMID: 33298746.

30. Dezfulian C, Orkin AM, Maron BA, Elmer J, Girotra S, Gladwin MT, Merchant RM, Panchal AR, Perman SM, Starks MA, van Diepen S, Lavonas EJ; American Heart Association Council on Cardiopulmonary, Critical Care, Perioperative and Resuscitation; Council on Arteriosclerosis, Thrombosis and Vascular Biology; Council on Cardiovascular and Stroke Nursing; Council on Quality of Care and Outcomes Research; and Council on Clinical Cardiology. Opioid-associated out-of-hospital cardiac arrest: distinctive clinical features and implications for health care and public responses: a scientific statement from the American Heart Association. *Circulation.* 2021;143(16):e836–e870. doi: 10.1161/CIR.0000000000000958. Epub 2021 Mar 8. PMID: 33682423.

31. Kariisa M, Patel P, Smith H, Bitting J. Notes from the field: xylazine detection and involvement in drug overdose deaths – United States, 2019. *MMWR Morb Mortal Wkly Rep.* 2021;70(37):1300–1302. doi: 10.15585/mmwr.mm7037a4. PMID: 34529640; PMCID: PMC8445380.

32. Harada MY, Lara-Millán A, Chalwell LE. Policed patients: how the presence of law enforcement in the emergency department

impacts medical care. *Ann Emerg Med.*
2021;78(6):738–748. doi: 10.1016/j.
annemergmed.2021.04.039. Epub 2021
Jul 29. PMID: 34332806.

33. Baker EF, Moskop JC, Geiderman JM,
Iserson KV, Marco CA, Derse AR; ACEP
Ethics Committee. Law enforcement and
emergency medicine: an ethical analysis.
Ann Emerg Med. 2016;68(5):599–607. doi:
10.1016/j.annemergmed.2016.02.013.
Epub 2016 May 4. PMID: 27157455.

34. Moreira M, Buchanan J, Heard K.
Validation of a 6-hour observation
period for cocaine body stuffers. *Am
J Emerg Med.* 2011;29(3):299–303. doi:
10.1016/j.ajem.2009.11.022. Epub 2010

Apr 24. PMID: 20825819; PMCID:
PMC3000892.

35. Arora A, Jain S, Srivastava A, Mehta M,
Pancholy K. Body packer syndrome.
J Emerg Trauma Shock. 2021;14(1):51–52.
doi: 10.4103/JETS.JETS_41_20. Epub 2021
Mar 23. PMID: 33911438; PMCID:
PMC8054804.

36. Prosser JM. Internal concealment of
xenobiotics. In: Nelson LS, Howland M,
Lewin NA, Smith SW, Goldfrank LR,
Hoffman RS. (eds.). *Goldfrank's Toxicologic
Emergencies*, 11th ed. McGraw Hill, 2019.
Accessed June 17, 2022. https://accessemer
gencymedicine.mhmedical.com/content
.aspx?bookid=2569&sectionid=210266329

Human Trafficking

Inkyu Kim and Hanni Stoklosa

Vignette

A 17-year-old male presents alone to the emergency department (ED) late at night with a complaint of right flank pain. He reports that he fell down the stairs and landed on his right side. He also has pain in his left upper back that is chronic from an injury while playing basketball, but offers no further detail. With registration, he reports not remembering the details of his address and that his legal guardian will come pick him up later.

On examination he has significant swelling with tenderness to palpation of the right chest wall.

X-ray reveals a non-displaced right-sided rib fracture as well as multiple age-indeterminate posterior rib fractures on the left.

Given the multiple fractures and atypical injury with an inconsistent story, you provide a private and safe setting for the patient and begin a conversation about abuse and say, "I educate all of my patients about exploitation and abuse because violence is so common in our society, and violence can have a big impact on our health, safety, and well-being."[1] You provide some education and review information about human trafficking and then ask, "Sometimes I can't fix the problem, but I can connect people to the services they need. Maybe you are in a situation that I can't keep a secret, maybe someone is hurting you, and I must tell someone about it, and maybe that will help you get what you really need."[2]

It turns out that he had run away from home due to domestic violence between his parents and has been working at a restaurant in return for room and boarding. He has been accruing increasing debt because he gets paid less than minimum wage and cannot keep up with his landlord's fees. Tonight, he was kicked in the ribs because he has not been able to work as efficiently due to his back spasms. He had also previously been beaten and injured his left upper back.

You treat his pain making sure he can breathe comfortably and make sure he does not have any other injuries. Prior to discharge, you pause as you suspect he is a victim of human trafficking.

- How can you protect this child from further exploitation?
- What resources can you give him?

Introduction

According to the United Nations, human trafficking is defined as "the recruitment, transportation, transfer, harboring or receipt of people by means of the threat or use of force or other forms of coercion, or abduction, of fraud, of deception, of the abuse of power or of a position of vulnerability or of the giving or receiving of payments or benefits to achieve the consent of a person having control over another person, for the purpose of exploitation. Exploitation shall include, at a minimum, the exploitation of the prostitution of others or other forms of sexual exploitation, forced labor or services, slavery, or practices similar to slavery, servitude or the removal of organs."[3]

The Action–Means–Purpose (AMP) model is a framework to further understand the definition of the crime of trafficking. The trafficker takes "action" by means of recruitment, harboring and transporting victims, and then employs a "means" of force, fraud or coercion for the "purpose" of exploitation through sex or labor trafficking.[4] Importantly, trafficking does not necessarily entail transportation, or movement across state or country lines; i.e., someone may be trafficked within one's own home, as occurs commonly in familial trafficking (trafficking by one's family member).

Labor Trafficking

Under the United States Trafficking Victims Protection Act (TVPA) of 2000 and subsequent amendments, labor trafficking is defined as "the recruitment, harboring, transportation, provision, or obtaining of a person for labor or services, through the use of force, fraud or coercion for the purpose of subjection to involuntary servitude, peonage, debt bondage or slavery."[5] Labor trafficking can occur anywhere, including but not limited to the following industries: restaurant, manufacturing, construction, transportation, agriculture, cleaning services, and landscaping.

Sex Trafficking

Sex trafficking, under the TVPA, is defined as the "recruiting, harboring, transporting, providing, obtaining, patronizing, or soliciting of an individual through the means of force, fraud, or coercion for the purpose of commercial sex," where commercial sex is defined as "any sex act on account of which anything of value is given to or received by any person."[5] Furthermore, minors under age 18 in commercial sex are considered victims of human trafficking regardless of use of force, fraud, or coercion.

Trafficking in Urban Areas

The literature on human trafficking is in its nascent stages, so comparative literature describing human trafficking differences between urban and rural contexts is scant.

The industries in which trafficking victims are exploited tend to be those that are underregulated and underpaid in a given location. So, while someone could be trafficked in agriculture in an urban setting, they may be more likely to be exploited in a marijuana grow house than a farm. According to limited evidence, trafficking survivors in rural and urban areas exhibit similarities in risk factors and warning signs they may display to clinicians.[6]

Given a relatively higher concentration of anti-trafficking services in urban settings, it may be possible that emergency clinicians working in urban settings can more readily connect their patients with resources.[7,8] However, given the higher population densities, it may be that more victims of trafficking are vying for these same resources. And urbanity is not a monolith; i.e., robust transportation infrastructures necessary to reach social services, which may be present in coastal major metropolitan areas, may be absent in Midwestern urban settings.[6] One study showed that urban-based service providers, including health professionals, were more likely to have knowledge of human trafficking.[6]

Risk Factors

Human trafficking can affect persons of any age, socioeconomic status, religion, nationality, race, or ethnicity. However, particular populations are more at risk of being exploited. Unequal power dynamics and increased dependence on basic needs lead to more vulnerability to human trafficking. Socioeconomic risk factors include poverty, homelessness, undocumented or unstable immigration status, recent migration, gang involvement, prior incarceration, and language barriers.[9] Marginalized and disadvantaged communities are particularly vulnerable due to structural inequities. Moreover, people of color, the LGBTQIA+ community, recently incarcerated, elderly, unaccompanied minors, and people with developmental delay and physical disability have been shown to be targeted for human trafficking.[10,11] Mental illness or substance use disorders are also highly intertwined with trafficked victims.[12] Furthermore, intersectional forms of abuse increase the risk of human trafficking. For instance, people experiencing intimate partner violence, child abuse and family dysfunction, or instability incur a higher risk.[13,14]

Red Flags and Indicators

Identifying patients suffering from human trafficking is difficult given unconscious biases clinicians may have as well as a victim's fears around disclosing and lack of knowledge of their exploitation.[12,15] Clinicians in the ED should be on the lookout for "red flags," i.e., a constellation of indicators that are suspicious for human trafficking. The following advice is based on extant literature and promising practices, but more research needs to be conducted to fully understand the clinical patterns of presentation of human trafficking.[16]

Trafficked individuals can exhibit abnormal behavior that could be mistaken for mental health issues. Patients may be anxious, fearful, depressed, submissive, and tense overall, particularly when bringing up law enforcement. Behaviors to look out for are poor eye contact, inconsistent and changing history, and being overly protective of their personal belongings.[13]

Clinicians should also be aware of interactions between patients and people accompanying them. One-sided power dynamics are usually present in relationships between traffickers and trafficked individuals, which may be noticeable in the clinical setting. More subtly, trafficking victims may be accompanied by individuals at a similar level of exploitation by the trafficker as a "minder." That individual is meant to be eyes and ears for the trafficker and report back, and may be the same age, gender, ethnicity, or race as the trafficked patient.[17] Patients experiencing trafficking may not be allowed to speak for themselves. Patients may be reluctant to articulate their full history in the presence of their guests. Constantly glancing nervously at their guest for corroboration or hesitation should be a red flag. Additionally, accompanied guests may be directly providing history or interjecting over key pieces of history and physical examination.[13,17]

Relatedly, clinicians should be aware that those experiencing trafficking may lack control over basic things, including their own insurance information, money for co-pay, or identification documents. Victims may carry few or no personal possessions. Furthermore, for trafficking victims who may be moved from one place to another, and/or for whom English is a second language, they may not know how they got from their place of work or shelter to the ED.[18] In inquiring directly, or via chart review, elements of a patient's living and working conditions may reveal they are unable to come and go as needed from work, are unpaid or poorly paid, working excessively long or unusual hours, restricted in their breaks, in large debt, and working in areas with high security measures. Other indicators of human trafficking include loss of sense of time and numerous inconsistencies in the story.[13,17]

A combination of poor living and working conditions as well as lack of regular access to healthcare lead to health problems that may present atypically to the ED, relative to similar patients of their demographics. For example, a young, otherwise healthy patient may present with a sequela of chronic nutritional deficiencies including anemia, neuropathy, thin skin, or hair. Unhygienic working conditions could lead to infestations with fungi, scabies, and lice. On physical examination, evidence of multiple bruising, lacerations, hematomas, unexplained trauma, old and new fractures, cigarette and scald burns are findings concerning for abuse in victims of human trafficking. Furthermore, patients may have evidence of environmental injury including chemical exposures and hypo- or hyperthermia.[14,17]

Health Implications of Human Trafficking

Victims of human trafficking are at higher risk of certain health risks given the nature of their work. Many come to the ED as a primary source of immediate and intermittent care. Providing high-quality medical care that addresses social determinants of health is an important part of caring for those experiencing trafficking.

Labor Trafficking

Health implications of labor trafficking include communicable diseases, environmental exposures, workplace trauma, and chronic musculoskeletal issues.

Intensive labor with lack of proper resources may lead to severe dehydration and malnutrition.

Trafficked persons can be at higher risk of infections in unhygienic environments in their housing or during transport, such as ocean voyages and long rides. Communicable diseases, particularly endemic diseases, may cause severe health problems. Depending on the type and location of their work, victims may have exposure to malaria, chagas, cysticercosis, toxoplasmosis, toxocariasis, trichomoniasis, tuberculosis, HIV, typhoid, and other communicable diseases.[11,19]

Environmental exposures are a large concern for labor trafficked individuals. For example, miners are at higher risk of exposure to asbestos and silicosis, agricultural workers are exposed to organophosphate poisoning, and workers in the seafood industry may be exposed to *Vibrio vulnificus*. Temperature-related injuries with lack of safety gear and long working hours may lead to heat exhaustion or heat stroke, burns, hypothermia, and frostbite.[11,18,20]

People experiencing labor trafficking may not have the safety measures needed to protect themselves from workplace injuries. Labor trafficked individuals confer a higher risk of traumatic amputation, head trauma, falls, extremity injuries, electrocution, lung injury, and heavy metal poisonings.[21] Notably, both males and females who experience labor trafficking may be subject to sexual violence.[22,23]

Finally, given the high intensity and long work hours, trafficked workers may suffer from non–life-threatening but debilitating chronic musculoskeletal issues. Poor ergonomics, poor training, and poor safety measures can lead to chronic back pain, neck pain, arthritis, carpal tunnel, headaches, and vision problems.

Sex Trafficking

Patients experiencing sex trafficking may have unique traumatic injury that may be inconsistent with their history. Genitourinary injuries, particularly lacerations, hematomas, and pain from forced sexual encounters may be present. Furthermore, clinicians should know that those experiencing sex trafficking may present with strangulation or restraint injuries.[24,25]

Patients are at higher risk of sexually transmitted infections such as HIV/AIDS, herpes, syphilis, gonorrhea, chlamydia, trichomonas, hepatitis, and molluscum contagiosum. Delay in treatment of any sexually transmitted infections may result in higher risk for pelvic inflammatory disease, disseminated gonococcemia, AIDS, and liver failure.[14,24,25]

Obstetrics-related health implications of sex trafficking include presentations for emergency contraception, lack of follow-up obstetrics care, and delayed care for ectopic pregnancy. Uniquely, forced tampon use or placement of other absorptive material in the vagina ("packing of the vagina") to hide menstruation in sex trafficked individuals may result in vaginal infections and possibly toxic shock syndrome.[14,24]

Approach to a Potential Victim

Trauma-Informed Care

Trauma-informed care is an approach to a patient's care that recognizes the pervasive nature of trauma in order to better support the health needs of patient who have experienced trauma.[26] First, the goal of a clinical encounter with a potentially trafficked person is never to induce disclosure of their experience or facilitate their "rescue." The goal is to provide education and resources to empower the potential victim.

Human trafficking controls every inch of a person's life. Even when well-intended, if an emergency clinician approaches a potential victim by focusing on getting them to disclose their trafficking experience or trying to rescue them, they further take away the victim's limited power and control.[27] In order to build rapport and trust, providers including physicians, nurses, technicians, and specialists should practice trauma-informed care to prevent re-traumatization. Trauma-informed care is an opportunity to approach a victim of trauma in a way that acknowledges that the patient's life situation – past and present – is instrumental in providing effective healthcare and healing.[17,28]

Providers can use the "PEARR" mnemonic (provide privacy, educate, ask, and respect and respond) to provide a trauma-informed approach to assist victims in health care settings. The tool is based on a universal education approach to educate patients about abuse, neglect, or violence instead of screening questions.[1]

Sensitive topics should be discussed alone and in a safe and private setting. The patient's physical and psychological safety should be considered in all interactions. Examples include asking whether they would like to have the room door shut and asking about their preferred pronouns. Biases and stereotypes and historical trauma should be recognized and addressed as well. Clinicians should then educate patients in a non-judgmental manner that normalizes discussions around trauma.[25]

Clinicians should ask questions in a way that is relevant to the clinical scenario and based on the current evidence-based tools and open an opportunity for potential victims to share their concerns.[29] Clinicians should avoid eliciting unnecessary details of trauma particularly with multiple similar questions asked by different clinicians. Interviews should be done alone if possible, as many people who experience human trafficking may be accompanied by traffickers as friends or family. To speak to the potential victim alone, emergency clinicians should work with their team to strategize the means that will be the least obvious to the person accompanying the patient. For example, the clinician may speak to them in the radiology suite, or have registration pull the accompanying person out of the room to assist with the registration process. Forceful separation of the individuals is rarely indicated, as it could lead to the trafficker preventing further contact with healthcare systems or result in the trafficked individual being injured or punished.

If a patient does not disclose victimization or declines assistance, then clinicians should respect their wishes and respond appropriately with resources as preferred by the patient. Decisions should always be made in collaboration with the patient and with full transparency to level the power differences between the staff and the patients seeking care.

Finally, patients should be empowered to recognize, build on, and be validated to believe in their own resilience and ability to heal from trauma. In some instances, trafficked persons may have severe emotional and physical reactions that can impede communication. Victims may have disassociation or depersonalization while interacting with healthcare clinicians.

It is important to note that while screening tools may be useful as a guide to identifying victims of human trafficking, the tool by itself, without the support and education of the whole healthcare team and without the proper environment or culture of trauma-informed care, is less effective.[30]

Use of Interpreter

According to the United Nations Trafficking in Persons Global Report, over 70% of victims identified by law enforcement in the Netherlands, Italy, and Germany are foreign nationals.[31] A 2019 Federal Bureau of Investigations study found that 43% of labor trafficking victims were foreign nationals residing outside the United States.[32] As such, clinicians should be mindful of using an interpreter as necessary to better facilitate conversation as well as build better rapport. In cases where the clinician suspects human trafficking, it is even more important to not use the accompanied guest as the interpreter, even if they insist on interpreting.

Protocol Development

Recognizing human trafficking and gathering appropriate resources requires health-system and clinician-level education, training, and resources. It is imperative that protocols be created in order to help clinicians develop a consistent response to victims of human trafficking that are embedded in responses to trauma and violence.[33] As many of the policies and procedures will require multidisciplinary support, a team of social work, case management, psychiatry, and if needed law-enforcement should guide their creation.

Health, Education, Advocacy, Linkage (HEAL) trafficking and Hope for Justice Protocol offers a toolkit to guide clinicians to create a human trafficking health care protocol.[34] Many of the steps are delineated below.

Safety Considerations

There are several considerations regarding a patient's safety while in the ED. Potentially trafficked individuals may be experiencing a spectrum of threats and violence including threats against their family and imminent harm to themselves or others. It is imperative to collaborate directly and make decisions together with the patient to avoid jeopardizing their safety. Well-intended but unwarranted or unilateral decisions may be dangerous to the victims. The presence of security may be triggering for individuals experiencing trafficking, as they may have had prior negative experiences with law enforcement or fear arrest or deportation. Emergency departments may register the patient under an alias if necessary. If there is active violence or threats of violence, hospital security should likely be involved. Relatedly, hospital security should also complete trainings related to human trafficking, including trauma-informed care trainings.

Patients Who Decline Assistance

Patients who decline assistance should not be pushed to receive further aid. Resources such as national human trafficking hotline numbers and where to find further information should be given as needed in accordance with the wishes of the patient. Information should also be given discreetly, if necessary, as preferred by the patient.

Forensic Evaluation

Forensic evaluation should be offered to patients who were sexually assaulted and also who are victims of human trafficking, as available. It is important to let the patient know that forensic evidence may be collected at the time of presentation but does not necessarily need to be used depending on the preference of the patient. Forensic evaluation should be done, if possible, by a trained forensics clinician, a sexual assault nurse examiner (SANE; in cases of sexual assault), or by clinicians who have been forensically trained. Examinations for sexual assault forensic evidence should ideally be done within 72 hours and be offered with full transparency that legal involvement may be needed depending on local mandated reporting laws.[35]

External Reporting and Documentation

Laws regarding human trafficking vary from state to state and nation to nation. Clinicians should know their local guidelines regarding mandated reporting. For instance, in the United States, some states have mandatory reporting for suspected human trafficking in minors. It is important to note that external reporting may violate the privacy of the patient; however, when required by law it can be done in a trauma-informed manner, sharing only the minimum data required.[36] If mandated reporting is necessary, as in the opening case, providers should be transparent about the limits of confidentiality prior to asking questions that could lead to a disclosure. Furthermore, if mandated reporting does occur, they can involve the patient in the reporting process as much as they would like to be (i.e., trauma-informed mandated reporting). Connection with local child welfare resources can be very helpful for coordination of the child's safe housing and safe transition out of their exploitative situation.

Resources

Resources should be obtained and distributed through multidisciplinary collaboration. In the United States there is a national hotline number for any trafficked persons to obtain resources and help. Additionally, depending on the situation and exploitation, and the patient's stated goals, further social and legal support should be provided. Follow-up appointments may be scheduled as a way to have consistent follow-up and for safety planning. Patients may be asked to follow-up with an outpatient social worker, outpatient medical clinic, or even be asked to return to the ED.

Challenges

Human trafficking is a hidden crime. Most victims often do not self-identify, and traffickers make it difficult for them to do so. Some people experiencing human trafficking may not perceive their exploitation as human trafficking depending on their cultural and national practices as well as their relationship to the traffickers (i.e., family members or loved ones).

Patients experiencing human trafficking may also be afraid of collateral damage if they receive assistance. Traffickers can threaten or harm the victim's family members, significant others, and the victims themselves if their exploitation is compromised. Trafficked individuals may be concerned about legal ramifications, such as their immigration status, or crimes committed during their trafficked work, such as selling drugs, stealing, and recruitment.

Many people experiencing human trafficking who are migrants are afraid of deportation even when they are legally in the United States, because they are unaware of their rights. Unstable or undocumented immigration status may be a barrier for victims to disclose their situation. For example, in the United States, as many as 67% of victims of labor trafficking are thought to be undocumented, and 28% thought to be in a "qualified alien status."[37] Many have precarious immigration status or have recently migrated and are unable or unwilling to communicate their full medical and complex social issues. Similarly, fear of unintended legal consequences such as being prosecuted for crimes committed during their captivity may hinder disclosure of their victimization.

Unconscious bias can prevent clinicians from "seeing" human trafficking, as the victim may not correspond to the clinician's stereotypes about what a trafficking victim looks like or how a victim may act. Additionally, due to the lack of awareness of how labor and sex trafficking presents to the ED, emergency clinicians may not identify trafficked individuals. The ED may represent the first place where someone experiencing trafficking is empowered with resources.

Vignette Conclusion

Having addressed his clinical issues, you share with him that based on what he has told you, what he is experiencing is a crime called human trafficking and that your ED is connected with resources that can help him. He says he is afraid for his life because his trafficker had threatened to kill him if he ever decided to quit. You remind him that you are mandated to report to the authorities regarding his exploitation as he is a minor (as you had mentioned earlier on in the visit) and give him the option to talk to social work to connect to resources or law enforcement. He refuses to speak to others, so you offer information about resources that he can take with him. You ask him if he would like the number to the human trafficking hotline or a brochure about it. He declines the brochure because he worries his trafficker might find it, but he enquires about the details of contacting the hotline. You confirm that he has a safe place to go at his uncle's home nearby and give him as much information as he requests and discharge him letting him know that the healthcare team is always here to help if he ever changes his mind, or he wants more information.

Pro-Tips

- Be aware of red flags and indicators of human trafficking, particularly unusual injuries that are inconsistent with a patient's history.
- Use interpreters for language barriers between clinicians and patients.
- Always strive to provide trauma-informed care.
- Be fully transparent and make decisions together with the patients experiencing human trafficking.
- Do not push patients to receive care or disclose.
- Create a health system protocol to combat human trafficking in order to provide consistent and efficient care to trafficked individuals.
- Assistance should be a multidisciplinary approach with social work, case management, local law enforcement, and other specialties as needed.
- Be aware of the intersectionality of human trafficking with other forms of abuse, such as intimate partner violence and child abuse.
- Understand your local legal mandates for reporting human trafficking.

References

1. HEAL Trafficking. PEARR Tool. 2021. https://healtrafficking.org/resources/pearr-tool/

2. Chisolm-Straker M, Baldwin S, Gaïgbé-Togbé B, Ndukwe N, Johnson PN, Richardson LD. Health care and human trafficking: we are seeing the unseen. *J Health Care Poor Underserved.* 2016;27 (3):1220–1233.

3. United Nations. Protocol to Prevent, Suppress and Punish Trafficking in Persons, Especially Women and Children, supplementing the United Nations Convention against Transnational Organized Crime. 2000. www.ohchr.org/en/instruments-mechanisms/instruments/protocol-prevent-suppress-and-punish-trafficking-persons

4. Polaris Project. Understanding the Definition of Human Trafficking: The Action–Means–Purpose Model. 2012.

5. Trafficking Victims Protection Act. 1469–1470. United States; pp. 106–386.

6. Schwarz C, Xing C, Daugherty R, Watt S, Britton HE. Frontline workers' perceptions of human trafficking: warning signs and risks in the Midwest. *J Hum Traffick.* 2020;6 (1):61–78. https://doi.org/101080/2332270520181562316

7. Bales K, Lize S. *Trafficking in Persons in the United States. A Report to the National Institute of Justice.* Croft Institute for International Studies, University of Mississippi,2005.

8. Cole J, Sprang G. Sex trafficking of minors in metropolitan, micropolitan, and rural communities. *Child Abuse Negl.* 2015;40:113–123.

9. Muraszkiewicz J. The tale of 400 victims: a lesson for intervention. *Arch Kryminol.* 2021;XLIII(1):75–96. Available from: https://czasopisma.inp.pan.pl/index.php/ak/article/view/2043

10. Toney-Butler TJ, Ladd M, Mittel O. Human trafficking. *StatPearls.* 2021 (accessed February 8, 2022). Available from: www.ncbi.nlm.nih.gov/books/NBK430910/

11. Knox S. Human Trafficking in America's Schools [Internet]. 2021. Available from: https://safesupportivelearning.ed.gov/sites/default/files/NCSSLE-2021HumanTraffickingGuide-508.pdf

12. Stoklosa H, MacGibbon M, Stoklosa J. Human trafficking, mental illness, and addiction: avoiding diagnostic overshadowing. *AMA J Ethics.* 2017;19 (1):23–34.

13. Tracy EE, MacIas-Konstantopoulos W. Identifying and assisting sexually exploited and trafficked patients seeking women's health care services. *Obstet Gynecol.* 2017;130(2):443–453.

14. Alpert EJ, Ahn R, Albright E, Purcell G, Burke TF, Macias-Konstantopolous W. *Human Trafficking: Guidebook on Identification, Assessment, and Response in the Health Care Setting.* Massachusetts Medical Society, 2014.

15. Chisolm-Straker M, Miller CL, Duke G, Stoklosa H. A framework for the development of healthcare provider education programs on human trafficking part two: survivors. *J Hum Traffick.* 2019;6 (4):410–424.

16. *Identifying Victims of Human Trafficking: What to Look for in a Healthcare Setting.* National Human Trafficking Resource Center, 2016.

17. Macias-Konstantopoulos W. Human trafficking: the role of medicine in interrupting the cycle of abuse and violence. *Ann Intern Med.* 2016;165 (8):582–588.

18. Stoklosa H, Kunzler N, Ma ZB, Luna JCJ, de Vedia GM, Erickson TB. Pesticide exposure and heat exhaustion in a migrant agricultural worker: a case of labor trafficking. *Ann Emerg Med.* 2020;76 (2):215–8.

19. Zimmerman C, Kiss L. Human trafficking and exploitation: a global health concern. *PLoS Med.* 2017;14(11). Available from: /p mc/articles/PMC5699819/

20. Marshall S, Taylor K, Connor T, Haines F, Tödt S. Will business and human rights regulation help Rajasthan's bonded labourers who mine sandstone? *J Indust Relat.* 2022;64(2):248–271. https://doi.org/ 10.1177/00221856211052073

21. Prakash J, Kim I, Erickson T, Stoklosa H. Migrant worker safety, occupational health equity, and labor trafficking. *Harvard Public Health Rev.* 2021;33.

22. Dank M, Farrell A, Zhang S, Hughes A, Abeyta S, Fanarraga I, Burke CP, Solis VO. An exploratory study of labor trafficking among U.S. citizen victims. *NCJRS* 302157; 2021.

23. Oram S, Abas M, Bick D, Boyle A, French R, Jakobowitz S, Khondoker M, Stanley N, Trevillion K, Howard L, Zimmerman C. Human trafficking and health: a survey of male and female survivors in England. *Am J Public Health.* 2016;106(6):1073–1078. Available from: https://ajph.aphapublications.org/doi/abs/ 10.2105/AJPH.2016.303095

24. Lederer LJ, Wetzel CA. The Health consequences of sex trafficking and their implications for identifying victims in healthcare facilities. *Ann Health Law.* 2014;23(1):61–91.

25. Shandro J, Chisolm-Straker M, Duber HC, Findlay SL, Munoz J, Schmitz G, Stanzer M, Stoklosa H, Wiener DE. Human trafficking: a guide to identification and approach for the emergency physician. *Ann Emerg Med.* 2016;68(4):501–508. Available from: www.annemergmed.com/ article/S0196064416300543/fulltext

26. Brown T, Ashworth H, Bass M, Rittenberg E, Levy-Carrick N, Grossman S, Lewis-O'Connor A, Stoklosa H. Trauma-informed care interventions in emergency medicine: a systematic review. *West J Emerg Med.* 2022;23(3):334–344.

27. Lewis-O'Connor A, Warren A, Lee J V., Levy-Carrick N, Grossman S, Chadwick M, Stoklosa H, Rittenberg E. The state of the science on trauma inquiry. *Womens Health (Lond Engl).* 2019;15:1745506519861234.

28. Trauma-Informed. *The Trauma Toolkit.* Klinic Community Health Centre, Winnipeg; 2013. www.trauma-informed.ca

29. Chisolm-Straker M, Singer E, Rothman EF, Clesca C, Strong D, Loo GT, Sze JJ, d'Etienne JP, Alanis N, Richardson LD. Building RAFT: trafficking screening tool derivation and validation methods. *Acad Emerg Med.* 2020;27(4):297–304.

30. Burns CJ, Runcie M, Stoklosa H. "We measure what we value": building the science to equitably respond to labor and sex trafficking. *Acad Emerg Med.* 2021;28 (12):1483–1484.

31. United Nations Office on Drugs and Crime. Global Report on Trafficking in Persons [Internet]. 2009. Available from: www.unodc.org/documents/human-trafficking/Global_Report_on_TIP.pdf

32. Human Traffickers Almost Certainly Engage in Sex Trafficking as Most Prevalent Form of Human Trafficking, Threatening Economic and Social Interests. 2019.

33. Tiller J, Reynolds S. Human trafficking in the emergency department: improving our response to a vulnerable population. *West J Emerg Med*. 2020;21(3):549–554.

34. Baldwin SB, Barrows J, Stoklosa H. *Protocol Toolkit for Developing a Response to Victims of Human Trafficking in Healthcare Settings*. HEAL Trafficking and Hope for Justice, 2017.

35. US Department of Justice. A National Protocol for Sexual Assault Medical Forensic Examinations. 2013.

36. Powell C, Asbill M, Brew S, Stoklosa H. Human trafficking and HIPAA: what the health care professional needs to know. *J Hum Traffick*. 2018;4(2):105–113. Available from: www.tandfonline.com/doi/abs/10.1080/23322705.2017.1285613

37. Banks D, Kyckelhahn T. *Characteristics of Suspected Human Trafficking Incidents, 2008–2010*. US Department of Justice, 2011.

Further Reading

1. International Labour Organization. Global Estimates of Modern Slavery Forced Labour and Forced Marriage [Internet]. International Labour Organization, 2017 (accessed February 7, 2022). Available from: www.ilo.org/wcmsp5/groups/public/@dgreports/@dcomm/documents/publication/wcms_575479.pdf

Travelers from Overseas

Arha Cho, Erena Weathers, and Geoffrey W. Jara-Almonte

Vignette

A man in his 20s presents to the emergency department (ED) complaining of four days of right upper quadrant abdominal pain. He reports traveling to Bangladesh 10 days prior where he had "food poisoning" with nausea and vomiting. He had onset of pain several days later, and today developed non-bloody diarrhea. Labs are remarkable for white blood cell count of 13. Stool studies are sent, and the patient is discharged. He returns to the ED 5 days later with fever, cough, and shortness of breath with resolved abdominal pain and diarrhea. Blood cultures are sent, a chest x-ray is normal, and a malaria screen is negative. He is again discharged with a diagnosis of viral syndrome.

He subsequently presents to another ED 2 days later complaining of right upper quadrant abdominal pain. AST is 612, ALT 577. A computed tomography (CT) scan of the abdomen reveals right lower quadrant adenopathy. He is admitted to the hospital.

- What disease entities must be considered?
- What additional diagnostic tests should be ordered?

Introduction

Urban centers serve as the major points of entry for those returning from international travel. Up to 8% of persons traveling from industrialized nations to the developing world report becoming ill enough to require medical care either during their travel or upon return.[1] Clinicians working in major urban travel hubs must be familiar with diseases endemic to foreign countries, emerging infectious threats, and with problems common to those who have traveled for the purpose of receiving medical care.

Care of the returning traveler can represent a conundrum for the busy urban emergency physician. Most patients who present following travel will have benign self-limited conditions that represent little risk to themselves or others. Nevertheless, some patients will present with serious illnesses or emerging infectious diseases that, if missed at initial presentation, may result in an avoidable adverse outcome for the patient or community. Many diseases acquired during travel have typical symptomatology and presentation that would be familiar to a physician practicing in an endemic area but represent a diagnostic challenge to clinicians who rarely see those conditions. Emergency clinicians are expected to maintain constant vigilance for these conditions among their multitude of other responsibilities.

General Approach

The first step in assessing any complaint in a traveler is recognizing that they have, indeed, recently traveled.

As with any ED encounter, the cornerstone of the evaluation of the returning traveler is securing an adequate history. Many patients may not offer a history of travel unless prompted, and even then, language and cultural barriers may add to the challenge. Once the emergency clinician recognizes that their patient has recently returned from abroad, it is worthwhile to slow down and take extra time to review details of the patient's travel itinerary, review diseases endemic to the area and any reported outbreaks.

Infectious diseases that commonly afflict returning travelers often have initially non-specific manifestations such as fever, myalgias, fatigue, headache, and gastrointestinal symptoms. It is imperative to consider these symptoms within the context of recent international travel. While a diagnosis of non-specific viral illness and routine primary care follow-up may be appropriate in other circumstances, for the ill returned traveler it is worthwhile to entertain a broader differential.

In addition to those who travel for business and leisure, the number of patients traveling abroad to secure medical care is common. Patients who have received care abroad and experience a complication will often present to urban EDs for further management. The clinician must be familiar with common procedures performed abroad, and be aware of potential complications.

Infectious Disease

Infectious diseases make up most complaints encountered in the returning traveler. Symptoms and signs are often nonspecific (such as fever) or attributable to involvement of the gastrointestinal and cutaneous systems.

Triage and Screening

On September 25, 2014, a traveler recently returned from Liberia visited an ED in Texas complaining of fever. He was evaluated and discharged only to return 3 days later, at which point he was diagnosed with Ebola virus and placed in isolation. He died 14 days later and two staff were infected. At that point there was a known Ebola outbreak and clinicians had been cautioned to remain vigilant for patients with suspicious signs or symptoms and a travel history. In review of this case it was determined that, while travel history was screened in triage, systems to implement rapid isolation of patients with the combination of concerning symptoms and travel history, or to ensure communication of essential information from triage team to treating clinicians, were not in place.[2]

Facilities should adopt a structured approach to identify patients with potential novel infectious diseases. Written signage should encourage patients to self-report travel and infectious symptoms. A travel screen at the initial registration or triage should seek to rapidly identify those who have traveled to areas with the potential for novel infectious threats and identify cardinal symptoms of infection. Screening protocols should consider current global outbreak sites and specific signs/symptoms of those diseases. Rapid isolation of those who screen positive and early use of infection prevention and control measures by staff may avoid spread.

Illnesses Characterized by Fever

Fever is a common presenting complaint in the returning traveler. In one retrospective study, over a quarter of patients returning from abroad cited fever as a reason for seeking care. Patients with fever were almost 9 times as likely to be hospitalized as those without.[3] The most common specific diagnoses assigned to those with fever are malaria and dengue followed by *Salmonella typhi*.

History

A patient returning from abroad with a fever must be subjected to screening questions on arrival. Determining location of travel is the most critical initial question; knowledge of regions visited will determine the most likely cause of fever (Table 6.1). For example, malaria is the most common cause of fever in returning travelers from Sub-Saharan Africa while dengue is the most common cause among those returning from Latin America or Asia. However, other concerning causes of fever in a returning traveler must also be screened, such as Ebola risk in patients returning from areas of outbreak. A quick screen to determine need for special isolation precautions for patients is important in the triage scenario of a febrile returning traveler.

In addition to determining location of travel, clinicians should ascertain which activities were participated in while abroad. Screening questions about water exposure, sexual activity, tattoos, medical care abroad, type of dwelling they stayed in, and use of nets can help determine the risk of exposure to illnesses endemic to the area in which they traveled. Asking about vaccination status prior to travel as well as medical prophylaxis during travel can help narrow down the differential for cause of fever.

Obtaining a thorough timeline of travel is important when trying to ascertain the cause of fever. Most tropical illnesses will manifest within a month of return, but there have been cases of malaria diagnosed greater than a year after inoculation. The clinician should solicit an accurate and thorough timeline of symptoms as well; this may assist in determining the probable incubation period, which will aid in diagnosis (Table 6.2).

As with other patients presenting with fever, a thorough review of systems should be conducted. It is unlikely that a patient will present with fever in isolation, so determining the other organ system involved or other characteristics of the fever can help with diagnosis. Identifying additional localizing symptoms will aid greatly in the diagnosis (Table 6.3). As always, the clinician needs to also think of common causes of fever, such as pneumonia, pyelonephritis, or viral upper respiratory infection (URI).

Table 6.1 Common Etiologies of Travel-Related Fever by Region

Caribbean/Central America	Chikungunya, dengue, Zika, malaria, leptospirosis, histoplansmosis, leishmaniasis
South America	Chikungunya, dengue, Zika, malaria, leptospirosis, histoplasmosis, enteric fever
Sub-Saharan Africa	Malaria, tickborne rickettsial infection, schistosomiasis, dengue, chikungunya, Ebola, Lassa
Southeast Asia	Dengue, malaria, chikungunya, leptospirosis, SARS
South-central Asia	Dengue, malaria, chikungunya

Table 6.2 Probably Etiology of Fever by Incubation Period

Incubation period < 10 days	Incubation period > 10 days	Variable incubation period
Dengue	Acute HIV	Malaria
Rickettsial infection	Acute schistosomiasis	Enteric fever
Chikungunya	Q fever	
Zika	Tuberculosis	
Leptospirosis	Visceral leishmaniasis	
	Brucellosis	

Table 6.3 Probable Etiology of Fever Based on Localizing Symptoms

Fever with abdominal pain/GI complaint	*Shigella, Salmonella*, ETEC, EHEC, pyogenic liver abscess, amebic liver abscess, cholera
Fever with respiratory complaint	COVID-19, influenza, SARS, MERS, tuberculosis, Hantavirus, histoplasmosis, Legionnaires
Fever with rash	Infected insect bites, cellulitis, lymphagitis, Rickettsial infections, leishmaniasis, filariasis, loiasis, HIV, measles, rubella
Fever with hemorrhage	Viral hemorrhagic fevers (Ebola, dengue, yellow fever, Lassa), spotted fever, leptospirosis
Fever with neurological complaint	Meningococcal meningitis, West Nile, rabies, tick borne encephalitis, cerebral malaria, polio
Fever with jaundice	Acute viral hepatitis, malaria, yellow fever, leptospirosis
Fever with eosinophilia	Acute schistosomiasis, *Strongyloides*, parasitic infections

COVID-19, coronavirus disease 2019; EHEC, enterohemorrhagic *Escherichia coli*; ETEC, enterotoxigenic *Escherichia coli*; GI, gastrointestinal; HIV, human immunodeficiency virus; MERS, Middle East Respiratory Syndrome; SARS, Severe Acute Respiratory Syndrome.

Physical Exam

A complete physical exam should be performed on all returning travelers presenting with fever. Attention should be paid to vital signs; tachycardia may be secondary to fever or suggestive of a more severe systemic inflammatory response. Response to antipyretics should be noted. If tachycardia persists after defervescence, another cause should be sought. Relative bradycardia in the setting of fever is a feature of *Salmonella enterica* infection. It is important to recall that the fever in malaria may wax and wane; as such, greater than 40% of patients may not have fever in the ED.[4] The clinician should look for scleral icterus, which may be seen in malaria, acute hepatitis, or dengue. Dry mucous membranes may suggest dehydration, potentially secondary to gastrointestinal losses. A pulmonary exam should evaluate for suggestions of pneumonia or pleural effusion. A thorough abdominal exam should be performed to ascertain evidence of tenderness or peritoneal inflammation, which may suggest enteric fever. A careful skin exam will reveal the presence of rashes. The neurological exam may reveal evidence of central nervous system involvement in the setting of malaria.

Precautions

As with any patient presenting to the ED, it is important to quickly assess if the febrile traveler is exhibiting signs or symptoms requiring urgent or emergent interventions. This assessment should be similar to routine rapid assessment involving airway, breathing, and circulation while also evaluating for signs of hemorrhage or neurological complication. It is also important to ascertain the need for special isolation precautions. Those presenting with hemorrhagic fevers such as Ebola or Lassa require strict barrier precautions, while those with respiratory complaints such as Middle East Respiratory Syndrome (MERS) or tuberculosis (TB) require airborne precautions and recommended N95 use. When in doubt about appropriate precautions in an ill returning traveler, the highest level of precaution is recommended and can be quickly de-escalated to the appropriate contact precaution.

Laboratory Studies

Routine laboratory studies including complete blood count, basic metabolic profile, liver enzyme, blood cultures, and urinalysis are recommended in returning travelers with fever. Laboratory abnormalities including acidosis, hypoglycemia, severe anemia, and elevated bilirubin may be seen in the setting of malarial infection. If travel history is suggestive, a malarial parasite screen should also be obtained. Hemorrhagic dengue fever is associated with marked thrombocytopenia. Abnormalities of liver enzymes and bilirubin levels may be seen in other conditions including viral hepatitis, liver abscess, yellow fever, leptospirosis, non-dengue hemorrhagic fevers, and cholangitis due to liver fluke infection. In the patient with fever and respiratory symptoms, attention should be paid to the eosinophil count, as peripheral eosinophilia is suggestive of parasitic infection including acute schistosomiasis, filariasis, roundworms such as *Ascaris*, strongyloidiasis, and fungal infections.

Differential Diagnosis, Treatment, and Disposition

Key considerations in returning travelers presenting with isolated fever or fever and non-specific symptoms is discussed below. Some of these conditions may present with localizing signs later in the course of illness, but early on there may be less information available to aid in a diagnosis.

Dengue

Dengue fever is a clinical syndrome caused by one of four flaviviruses transmitted by *Aedes aegypti* and *A. albopictus*. *A. aegypti* appears to be the primary vector; areas of high-risk for dengue mirror those in which *ageypti* is most prevalent, including Central and South America, the Caribbean Islands, Sub-Saharan Africa and South Asia, Southeast Asia, and the Pacific Islands. Cases have been reported in the southern United States as well.

Infection with any one serotype leads to long-term immunity against reinfection with the same serotype. Primary infection also leads to production of antibodies with cross-reactivity across all dengue serotypes. These antibodies will provide short-term immunity; however, as effectiveness wanes reinfection with other serotypes becomes possible. At lower concentrations the presence of these cross-reacting antibodies serves to paradoxically increase cellular virus uptake if reinfection occurs – termed antibody-dependent enhancement – and increases the risk for severe disease.

The clinical spectrum of dengue may range from mild infection to severe septic shock. The initial febrile phase lasts three to five days and is characterized by sudden onset of high fever and non-specific symptoms including headache, vomiting, myalgias, and transient rash. Hemorrhagic manifestations including petechiae and mucosal bleeding may be seen in this phase, although they are rarely severe. Following the febrile phase most patients recover; however, some develop a syndrome of severe capillary leak resulting in peritoneal and pleural fluid accumulation, intravascular volume depletion, and shock that may be accompanied by severe hemorrhagic complications. This is termed the critical phase and lasts 24–48 hours. The 2009 World Health Organization (WHO) classification (Figure 6.1) aids in risk-stratifying patients and guiding disposition and treatment.[5]

A tetravalent dengue vaccine – CYD-TDV (Dengaxia) – was approved in 2021 for use in patients aged 9–16 with serologic evidence of prior dengue infection who live in an endemic area. Vaccination is contraindicated in the absence of evidence of prior infection due to the risk of antibody-dependent enhancement.

Treatment of severe dengue infection is supportive. Healthy patients with primary infection, no warning signs, and close outpatient follow-up may be managed as outpatients. Inpatient management is warranted for others. Close monitoring for signs of extravascular fluid accumulation is warranted for those at risk of dengue shock; in general, this will occur between days 3 and 7 of illness, and may develop rapidly. WHO treatment protocols recommend initial crystalloid followed by colloid if there is failure to improve, or blood product replacement if low/falling hematocrit.

Malaria

Malaria should be considered in all travelers who present with fever or history of fever returning from areas in which malaria is endemic. The fever in malaria tends to be intermittent, and so many patients will present afebrile. Earlier in the disease process febrile paroxysms will happen irregularly; however, in later stages the release of parasites from erythrocytes becomes synchronous, leading to the classic cyclical fever. With earlier diagnosis, this presentation of cyclical fever has become uncommon, although it is worth recalling that every other day fevers are characteristic of disease caused by *Plasmodium falciparum* and *P. vivax*. Diagnosis can be established by visualization of the parasites on the thick and thin blood smears or by rapid parasitological testing.

Patients with suspected severe malarial disease should have treatment initiated as soon as possible. This group includes patients with proven or suspected *P. falciparum* parasitemia and evidence of impaired consciousness, convulsions, acidosis, hypoglycemia, severe anemia, renal impairment, jaundice, pulmonary edema, significant bleeding, shock, or hyperparasitemia (*P. falciparum* > 10%). Intravenous therapy with artesunate is preferred; this drug was approved by the Food and Drug Administration (FDA) in 2020 and is now commercially available. The dose is 2.4 mg/kg/dose, given at 0, 12, and 24 hours. If intravenous artesunate is not available then treatment with an oral medication such as artemether-lumefantrine, atovaquone-proguanil, quinine, or mefloquine is acceptable until it is possible to procure artesunate. If artesunate is not available locally, it can be obtained from the Centers for Disease Control and Prevention (CDC). The CDC maintains a malaria hotline (staffed during business hours) and a malaria clinician is on call who can provide consultation on diagnosis and treatment. Contact information can be found in their malaria

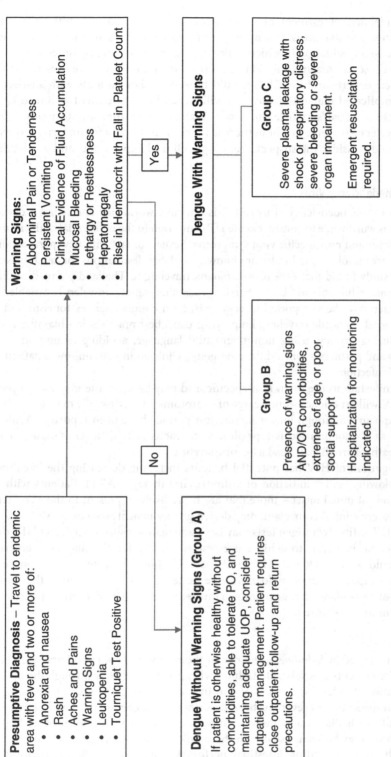

Presumptive Diagnosis – Travel to endemic area with fever and two or more of:
- Anorexia and nausea
- Rash
- Aches and Pains
- Warning Signs
- Leukopenia
- Tourniquet Test Positive

Warning Signs:
- Abdominal Pain or Tenderness
- Persistent Vomiting
- Clinical Evidence of Fluid Accumulation
- Mucosal Bleeding
- Lethargy or Restlessness
- Hepatomegaly
- Rise in Hematocrit with Fall in Platelet Count

No

Yes

Dengue With Warning Signs

Dengue Without Warning Signs (Group A)

If patient is otherwise healthy without comorbidities, able to tolerate PO, and maintaining adequate UOP, consider outpatient management. Patient requires close outpatient follow-up and return precautions.

Group B

Presence of warning signs AND/OR comorbidities, extremes of age, or poor social support

Hospitalization for monitoring indicated.

Group C

Severe plasma leakage with shock or respiratory distress, severe bleeding or severe organ impairment.

Emergent resuscitation required.

Figure 6.1 Approach to dengue – World Health Organization 2009 Guidelines.

treatment guidelines.[6] Treatment of uncomplicated malaria may be initiated with oral medication after the diagnosis has been confirmed. Infectious disease consultation is recommended in any situation in which malarial treatment is being considered.

Patients with severe malaria should be admitted to an intensive care unit and consultation with local experts and the CDC should be sought. For patients with suspected or proven uncomplicated malaria disposition will depend on the patient's clinical appearance, risk factors, social support, and ready availability of appropriate follow-up. For returning travelers with fever in whom there is no clinical concern for malaria, disposition decisions should consider the suspected etiology, clinical appearance, and availability of follow-up.

Human Immunodeficiency Virus

While human immunodeficiency virus (HIV) is endemic worldwide and is not a disease of travel *per se*, it is worthwhile to consider acute HIV infection in the differential of the returning traveler with fever and non-specific viral symptoms. Sexual contact with new partners during travel is not uncommon. Some locales are known as global destinations for sex tourism; for example, one study found that 66% of Australians traveling to Thailand planned on having a sexual encounter while abroad.[7] Use of barrier precautions among travelers is variable.[8] Both men and women have been reported to engage in both commercial sex tourism and non-commercial casual sex while traveling. Employing usual best practices in obtaining a sexual history – ensuring privacy, using non-judgmental language, avoiding assumptions about sexual activity and partners – will aid the emergency clinician in determining a patient's risk for acute HIV infection.

While manifestations are often non-specific and may be mild, the majority of patients with acute HIV will experience some degree of symptoms.[9] These usually manifest within 2–4 weeks of exposure, although longer incubation periods have been reported. Acute HIV may present as a mononucleosis-type illness characterized by fever, fatigue, malaise, lymphadenopathy, sore throat, headache, or diarrhea.

Early recognition of HIV has potential benefits including decreasing the likelihood of spread and allowing earlier initiation of antiretroviral therapy (ART). Patients with more severe symptoms at initial onset – those that are more likely to present to the ED – tend to have a more severe clinical course and may derive greater benefit from early ART.

Modern HIV antibody/antigen tests may have adequate sensitivity to detect HIV during the acute viremia; however, to achieve greatest sensitivity for the diagnosis emergency clinicians should also check the HIV viral load. During the acute viremic phase viral reproduction is rapid and the viral load may be quite high. In most facilities the results of this test will not be available in time to inform immediate treatment decisions, and so careful follow-up planning is required.

Enteric Fever

Enteric fever is caused by *Salmonella enterica* of the serotypes Typhi and Paratyphi. Enteric fever classically presents in a subacute fashion with progressive fever through the first week of illness followed by development of abdominal pain during the second week. Relative bradycardia in the setting of fever has been described. Both constipation and diarrhea may be present, although diarrhea is more common. A truncal rash described as "salmon-colored" macules may be seen, usually on the trunk and abdomen. During the third week severe complications including intestinal perforation may occur. Bowel perforation is thought to be due to hyperproliferation of Peyer's patches at the ileocecal junction. The exact frequency of this complication is unknown but has been reported to be as high as 10%; mortality is high.[10,11]

Enteric fever should be considered in the patient with fever who has recently traveled to an endemic area. Most cases diagnosed in the US are associated with travel to South Central and Southeast Asia.[12] Diarrhea, constipation, and abdominal pain should increase suspicion for the diagnosis; their absence is not reassuring in the early stages of disease. Blood and stool cultures should be taken although yields have been reported as low as 50% and 30% for blood and stool, respectively. Bone marrow cultures have the highest sensitivity but are rarely performed in clinical practice. Enteric fever is vaccine preventable; patients traveling from resource-rich countries to endemic areas should have received pre-travel immunization.

For patients with known or suspected enteric fever, oral or parenteral treatment may be chosen depending on disease severity. Fluoroquinolones or macrolides may be used as oral therapy, while second- and third-generation cephalosporins or carbapenems may be used for parenteral treatment. Corticosteroids might reduce mortality and should be considered as adjuvant therapy in patients with severe systemic illness. Perforation, if present, requires prompt surgical referral. As of 2022, travel to Iraq and Pakistan was associated with higher risk of infection with an extensively drug-resistant strain and broader-spectrum treatment recommended for patients with a history of travel to these locations.[13]

Chikungunya

Chikungunya virus is a mosquito-borne virus that presents with fever. It is endemic to West Africa, and sporadic outbreaks have occurred across the tropics including the Caribbean. Cases of local transmission have been reported in Florida. Most cases diagnosed in the United States have been in patients with recent travel to the Caribbean including the Dominican Republic, Puerto Rico, and Haiti.

The incubation period ranges from 1 to 14 days, with most patients becoming symptomatic by 7 days. Symptoms include fever with predominant arthralgias and myalgias. Arthralgias may precede fever and may be associated with synovitis and acute joint effusions. The acute febrile episode is generally resolved within 3–5 days; however, musculoskeletal complaints may persist for weeks to months after the initial illness.

Severe complications have been reported but are rare and more often occur in patients at the extremes of age. Therapy is supportive with no specific disease treatments available.

Zika

Similar to dengue, zika is a mosquito-borne flava virus first encountered in Uganda in 1947 that has subsequently been encountered throughout the tropics. Significant outbreaks have occurred in the Caribbean and Latin America. The major clinical concern with Zika infection is its association with fetal abnormalities, particularly congenital microcephaly.

Manifestations of Zika are non-specific and include fever (usually low grade) arthralgias, myalgias, and rash. Only 20–25% of cases are symptomatic. Zika may be transmitted through sexual contact.

Because of its effect on pregnancy, emergency clinicians will most frequently encounter returned travelers who are concerned that they or a partner may have encountered the virus. Women who present after traveling to a Zika-endemic area should have a pregnancy test performed. Symptomatic patients may receive polymerase chain reaction (PCR) testing on whole blood or urine within 7 days of symptom onset. Testing is not recommended for non-pregnant asymptomatic individuals. The decision to test asymptomatic pregnant women is controversial and is not recommended by the CDC.[14]

Diarrheal Illnesses

Acute diarrhea is defined as the passage of unusually loose stools lasting <14 days. Among all returning travel patients who seek medical care, acute unspecified diarrheal illness was the most common specific diagnosis provided.[15] The majority of diarrhea cases presenting to the ED do not require significant workup; conservative management at home usually suffices. This can be applied as well to the well returning traveler whose complaint is diarrhea without other associated symptoms. If this patient appears well without signs of dehydration, the management is similar to non-traveler patients with the same complaint. One medication to recommend to patients experiencing uncomplicated traveler's diarrhea is bismuth salicylate or loperamide to help with symptoms. Loperamide is not to be used in those with bloody diarrhea.

History

The history should focus on determining acuity of diarrhea, timing of onset in relation to associated symptoms, and the character of diarrhea. Simultaneous onset of vomiting and diarrhea may suggest a bacterial exotoxin as opposed to an invasive pathogen. Quantity of diarrheal stools may help differentiate a secretory process from an inflammatory or invasive one. Large-volume watery stools are more associated with secretory diarrhea as opposed to invasive disease, which is characterized by frequent small-volume stools with associated tenesmus. Inquiry should be made into the presence of associated blood or mucus. While the odor of diarrhea is seldom pleasant, particularly malodorous diarrhea and flatulence is associated with *Giardia* infections. The clinician should inquire about associated symptoms including abdominal pain, fever, and rash.

In addition to a standard history and physical, the clinician should obtain a thorough travel history including locations to which the patient traveled and activities in which they engaged. Ask about contact with animals, consumption of undercooked meat, encounters with contaminated water, and any wilderness travel. It is surprising how often high-risk activities may be overlooked if they are not expressly queried.

Physical Exam

The clinician should use the physical exam to determine the patient's overall clinical status, identify dehydration, assess for evidence of invasive organisms, and evaluate for signs of specific pathogens or severe complications of diarrheal illness. Dehydration is a significant risk in severe diarrhea and it is worth remembering that, despite the relatively benign clinical course of diarrheal illnesses in the United States, worldwide diarrhea is a leading cause of death. Careful attention should be paid to signs of dehydration including skin turgor and mucous membranes. Severe dehydration leaving to impaired perfusion may manifest with delayed capillary refill, thready pulse, and metabolic acidosis with compensatory hyperpnea.

Children – infants in particular – are exceptionally susceptible to volume loss from diarrhea; if their premorbid weight is known, then an accurate assessment of volume depletion can be made by weighing them at the emergency visit. The degree of weight lost can be used to assess degree of dehydration. Severe dehydration is associated with decreased activity, listlessness, and lethargy. In the patient with open fontanelles an assessment of their fullness should be made. Every fontanelle is a little different, so asking the parents if it seems abnormal is helpful.

In addition to assessing hydration status the clinician should perform a thorough abdominal exam. Evidence of organomegaly should be sought and tenderness should be noted. A rash, if present, may suggest a causative organism. Salmon-colored macules may be seen later in the course of *Salmonella typhi* infection, whereas petechiae and purpura are worrisome for hemolytic uremic syndrome (HUS) secondary to Shiga toxin producing *Escherichia coli* or *Shigella dysenteriae*.

Differential Diagnosis

Traveler's Diarrhea

This is the most common affliction of travelers venturing from resource-rich to resource-poor settings; 40–60% of such travelers will experience diarrhea.[16] It is usually self-limited and benign. Typical etiologies are enterotoxigenic or enteroaggregative *E. coli* (ETEC), although viruses and *Shigella* or *Campylobacter* species may cause a similar syndrome. Typical symptoms are abdominal cramping, fatigue, malaise, low-grade fever, and sudden onset of watery diarrhea. It is not associated with blood or pus in the stool.

Symptoms typically begin within the first 2 weeks of arrival and last 1–5 days. A small minority of patients will experience symptoms lasting longer than a week. Treatment is generally supportive, although antibiotics are often prescribed; they may decrease duration of symptoms at the cost of promoting resistance, increasing risk of infection by resistant organisms, *Clostridium difficile* infection, and drug-associated adverse effects. Symptomatic treatment with antimotility agents or bismuth may be recommended for non-severe cases; probiotics may offer some benefit as well.

Giardia

Giardia lamblia (also referred to as *G. intestinalis or G. duodenalis*) is a protozoan parasite that occurs throughout the world and is a common cause of non-dysenteric diarrhea. Travelers become infected through consumption of contaminated water, food, or direct fecal–oral transmission. Wilderness travel, and in particular drinking unfiltered or untreated surface water, is a classic risk factor. Sexual contact is another important route of spread; any history of anal–oral contact should be sought.

Giardia trophozoites localize to the proximal small bowel. While they do not cause invasive infection, they attach to intestinal epithelium and may cause functional abnormalities leading to malabsorption.

Patients with acute giardiasis present with diarrhea that will often be described as greasy or particularly foul smelling, usually within 7–14 days of infection. Travel to Eastern Europe should raise suspicion for *Giardia*. The condition is associated with a higher incidence of upper gastrointestinal complaints than typical traveler's diarrhea including abdominal bloating and belching as compared to other causes of non-dysenteric diarrhea. Fatigue, malaise, and weight loss may also be present. Fever is rare.

Although less likely to be encountered in the emergency setting, *Giardia* may also establish a chronic infection resulting in loose stools without overt diarrhea and symptoms attributable to malabsorption including fatigue and stunted growth in children.

Nucleic amplification or antigen testing may be used to establish the diagnosis. These methods may have increased sensitivity compared to stool microscopy. Giardiasis may be prevented by avoidance of contaminated food and water. Drinking water should be boiled for at least 1 minute, filtered or treated with iodine or another method demonstrated to kill *Giardia* cysts.

Cholera

Cholera is characterized by acute secretory diarrhea caused by exotoxins produced by the bacterium *Vibrio cholerae*. Cholera has a short incubation period ranging from several hours to 5 days. Clinical deterioration may occur rapidly, usually within 24 hours of onset of symptoms. Transmission usually occurs via ingestion of unclean water or consumption of uncooked seafood. Person-to-person transmission may occur. Assessing the risk of cholera requires a thorough travel and exposure history – travel to a cholera-endemic area or site of an active outbreak, exposure to brackish water, or consumption of undercooked shellfish should raise suspicion.

In contrast to most causes of watery diarrhea, cholera is associated with high mortality rates of 10% to 48% if untreated.[17] Death is the result of severe volume depletion and electrolyte imbalances that occur due to the massive diarrhea. Clinical decompensation may occur rapidly after onset of diarrheal symptoms. In the case of patients presenting with severe cholera, diagnosis will likely be presumptive based on the history. Antigen testing is available, but depending on institutional availability may not be available in time to guide management of the critically ill patient.

The mainstay of therapy is volume resuscitation and electrolyte repletion. In resource-limited settings rehydration is often initiated with oral rehydration solution; however, for the urban clinician in a resource-rich setting, early intravenous therapy is warranted if cholera is suspected. Volume loss may be as rapid as 10–20 mL/kg/hour. Total volume required may be as high as 200–350 mL/kg over the first 24 hours, and volume loss over the course of illness may reach 1000 mL/kg. It is important to use isotonic crystalloid in the initial resuscitation, lactated Ringers may be a good choice as it contains both potassium and bicarbonate which are rapidly lost in acute secretory diarrhea. Antibiotics may shorten the duration of illness and reduce stool volume. Macrolides and fluoroquinolones have good activity against *V. cholerae*. Both can prolong the QTc interval, and care should be taken to monitor electrolytes closely.

Acute Dysentery

Dysentery is a clinical syndrome characterized by frequent but small-volume bloody diarrhea, and systemic signs and symptoms including fever, abdominal cramps, and tenesmus. Usually, this syndrome can be differentiated from acute watery diarrhea based on the history and physical exam, although symptoms may overlap. Dysentery may resemble acute gastroenteritis with acute nausea, vomiting, and diarrhea early in its course. Worldwide the most common etiology of dysentery is *Shigella*; other causes include enteroinvasive and enterohemorrhagic strains of *E. coli*, non-typhoidal *Salmonella*, *Campylobacter*, *Entamoeba*, and schistosomiasis.

Identifying dysentery has clinical relevance, as there are complications associated with common causative organisms. Shiga toxin producing *Shigella*, and *E. coli* can cause the hemolytic–uremic syndrome. Sepsis and bacteremia may occur with any invasive bacterial organism, but particularly *Salmonella* and *Shigella*. Neurological complications are also reported, including Guillain–Barré syndrome due to *C. jejuni* and seizures associated with *Shigella*. Enteric fever due to *Salmonella typhi* is another important cause of fever and abdominal pain that may be associated with diarrhea; differentiating this from other causes of dysentery is relevant due to the high mortality rate and need for early antibiotic therapy.

Diagnostic Testing

It is sometimes important to engage diagnostic tools when evaluating traveler's diarrhea. Infectious Disease Society of America (IDSA) guidelines recommend that stool testing should be performed for patients with diarrhea that is accompanied by fever, bloody and/ or mucoid stools, severe abdominal cramping, tenderness, or signs of sepsis.[18] This testing should involve testing for *Salmonella*, *Shigella*, *Campylobacter*, *Yersinia*, *C. difficile*, and Shiga-toxin producing *E. coli* (STEC). If a traveler is presenting with diarrhea of large volumes or "rice water" diarrhea and exposure to salty or brackish waters, consumption of raw or undercooked shellfish, or travel to cholera-endemic regions, then testing for *Vibrio* species is warranted. Testing is also recommended if the diarrhea lasts for longer than 14 days, and should involve testing for amebic causes such as *Giardia*.

Treatment

Empiric antimicrobial therapy for diarrheal illnesses is controversial. For acute watery diarrhea associated with travel, antibiotics may be considered. Treatment for traveler's diarrhea has been shown to decrease symptom duration; however, it is associated with various risks including promotion of drug resistance and adverse drug reactions.[19,20] Single-dose therapy is as effective as 3-days for traveler's diarrhea due to non-invasive pathogens, which is the majority of cases. There is equal efficacy between using fluoroquinolones versus azithromycin in most cases of traveler's diarrhea, but there has been increasing fluoro-quinolone resistance in Southeastern Asia so that azithromycin therapy is the recommended first line. Options for antibiotic therapy are outlined in Table 6.4.

Oral treatment of acute giardiasis typically resolves symptoms within one week. Failure to respond symptomatically may require treatment with an alternative regimen for combination therapy. Options for initial therapy include a single dose of tinidazole, 3 days of nitazoxanide, or a week of metronidazole. Albendazole and mebendazole are alternative agents.

In well-appearing immunocompetent patients presenting with bloody diarrhea to the ED, it is not recommended to administer empiric antibiotics while awaiting the results of their workup. Treatment of STEC strains such as O157 and others may increase the risk of developing HUS. In the case of the returning traveler with documented fever (temperature

Table 6.4 Treatments Options for Traveler's Diarrhea

Ciprofloxacin	500mg PO	3-day course
	750mg PO	Single dose
Levofloxacin	500mg PO	Single dose, 3-day course if not improved with single dose
Ofloxacin	400mg PO	Single dose, 30day course if not improved with single dose
Azithromycin	1000mg PO	Single dose
	500mg PO	3-day course
Rifaximin	200mg PO TID	3-day course

greater than 38.5 C) or other signs of sepsis associated with bloody diarrhea, it may be reasonable to begin empiric antibiotic therapy.[18]

Disposition

Acute diarrheal illness can generally be managed in the outpatient setting. Patients should have follow-up arrangements made with a primary care physician and be advised of any test results – such as stool culture – that are pending at the time of discharge. Clinicians should provide discharge instructions for oral hydration and discuss return precautions.

For those with watery diarrhea indications for admission include moderate dehydration that is not responding to oral hydration strategies, severe dehydration, electrolyte imbalances, and inability to tolerate oral intake regardless of hydration status. Children and especially infants with acute watery diarrhea are at increased risk of dehydration and have a low threshold for admission or observation. Consider admission for any patient with suspected cholera, given the rapidity with which severe symptoms may develop. Ill-appearing patients with signs of sepsis, bloody diarrhea, abdominal pain, and tenderness should be admitted, as should those with suspected complications related to acute dysentery such as HUS, seizures, or other neurological sequelae.

Emerging Infectious Threats

Assessing the returning traveler with signs or symptoms of infection must always include a consideration of emerging infectious diseases. Emergency clinicians must make themselves aware of ongoing outbreaks and familiarize themselves with the signs and symptoms of potential emerging threats. The CDC maintains a list of countries with active travel warnings; this resource should be readily available to clinicians in the ED for easy reference.

· Some concerning emerging and re-emerging infectious threats are summarized in Table 6.5. In addition, the viral hemorrhagic fevers (VHF) deserve special note. Several diseases have been identified which cause a severe illness characterized by a viral prodrome followed by severe immune activation, systemic inflammation, and progression to shock, multiorgan dysfunction, and death. Mortality rates are generally high. Hemorrhagic manifestations – although the namesake of these illnesses – are variable and are rarely the primary pathogenic process. A summary of VHF is provided in Table 6.6.

The single most important thing an emergency clinician can do to recognize a patient at risk of a novel infectious disease is obtain a thorough travel history.

That being said, the pitfalls of relying on a travel history to identify those at potential risk of novel infections were made clear by the coronavirus disease 2019 (COVID-19) pandemic. Widespread community transmission was likely occurring in urban areas such as New York City quite early in the pandemic, while screening efforts focused only on those with a travel history. Urban clinicians should assume that any emerging global threat that seems to exhibit direct person-to-person transmission can be spreading in their city.

Medical Tourism

According to one industry group, around 2.1 million Americans sought health care around the world in 2019 as part of a $74 billion global market for cross-border healthcare. While comprehensive data on destinations, services, and complications are unavailable, many of

Table 6.5 Emerging and Re-Emerging Infectious Diseases

Pathogen	Endemic region	Sign and symptoms	Prevention/ treatment
Plague	Worldwide	May present as febrile lymphadenitis (bubonisc) with localized painful lymoh bodes, severe systemic illness (septicemic) with or without localizing signs/symptoms, or sudden onset cough, hemoptysis, and chest pain (pneumonic	Aminoglycosides, fluoroquinolones, and doxycycline are all effective
Monkeypox	Central and West Africa	Initially fever and viral syndrome, followed by development of rash evolving from macules to vesicles to pustules over several weeks	Smallpox vaccine is effective in prevention, antivirals also available
Coronavirus	Worldwide	Initially fever and viral syndrome, followed by development of rash evolving from macules to vesicles to pustules over several weeks	Smallpox vaccine is effective in prevention, antivirals also available
Nipah virus	Malaysia, India, Bangladesh, Philippines	Sudden-onset fever, headache, and myalgias. Rapid progession of encephalitis syndrome with seizures, focal neurological deficits, and coma. Mortality rate of 30–90%	Supportive care
Measles	Worldwide	Fever, malaise, and cough followed by characteristic exanthem. May result in gastrointestinal, neurological and pulmonary complications	Vaccine preventable

these patients, referred to as "medical tourists," are low-income, vulnerable members of minority groups without adequate health insurance seeking affordable healthcare alternatives. Popular destinations include India, Thailand, China, and Latin America, and include procedures such as cosmetic surgeries and organ transplant.[21]

Cosmetic Surgery

According to a review study assessing the impact of surgical tourism, women dominate the cosmetic surgical market with 86.2% or roughly 20 million cosmetic procedures worldwide. Silicone implant breast augmentation surgery is the most common, followed by liposuction and eyelid surgery.[22] Gender-affirming surgery has been a small but increasing component of the cosmetic surgery and medical tourism industry. Thailand has emerged as the popular overseas destination for patients seeking gender-affirming surgery.[23] While countries outside the US can offer substantial savings in procedure costs, they are associated with hidden

Table 6.6 Viral Hemorrhagic Fevers

Pathogen	Reservoir/ vector	Endemic region	Signs and symptoms	Prevention/ treatment
Ebola (filovirus)	Unknown, possibly bats	Central Africa	Abrupt-onset fevers/chills followed by diarrhea. Variable rash. Mucosal bleeding noted later in disease process. Conjunctival injection and uveitis noted as well. Development of severe electrolyte abnormalities and disseminated intravascular dissemination	Multiple vaccine products and antibody-based therapies approved
Lassa fever (arenavirus)	African common rat (*Mastomeys*)	West Africa	Fever and malaise followed by non-specific symptoms. May progress to facial swelling, pulmonary edema, and mucosal bleeding. Mortality rate ~1% deafness in a common complication	Ribavirin may be effective if given within 6 days of onset of symptoms
Marburg (filovirus)	Egyptian fruit bat	Central and East Africa, primarily Uganda	Rapid onset of fevers/chills followed by weakness and anorexia. Vomiting and diarrhea may be present. Shock may develop. Mild petechial and mucosal bleeding may develop, usually not severe until end stages	Supportive care
Crimean– Congo	*Hyalomma* tick	Africa, southern	Sudden onset of fever, headache,	Supportive care

Table 6.6 (cont.)

Pathogen	Reservoir/ vector	Endemic region	Signs and symptoms	Prevention/ treatment
hemorrhagic fever (*Nairovirus*)		and Eastern Europe, Middle East	myalgias, abdominal pain, and vomiting, Mucosal, petechial, pulmonary, and intra-abdominal bleeding seen in severe cases	
Lujo hemorrhagic fever (arenavirus)	Unknown, presumed rodent	Single cluster described in South Africa	Onset of fatigue, malaise, and fever followed by nausea and vomiting, chest pain, and sore throat. A diffuse rash and facial swelling reported followed by neurologic deterioration and multi-organ failure	Ribavirin was given to the single survivor of the index cluster
South American hemorrhagic fever (various New World arenaviruses)	Rodents	South America	Five different arenaviruses reported. Incubation period of 3–21 days then fever and non-specific viral illness. This is followed by gastrointestinal symptoms, conjunctivitis, and mucosal bleeding. May develop neurological symptoms, severe hemorrhagic complications, shock, multi-organ failure and death	Vaccine for Jumin virus/Argentinian hemorrhagic fever. Convalescent plasma and ribavirin reported

expenses and complications that may not be immediately recognized, stemming from barriers in communication, lack of regulation, legal recourse, and global antibiotic resistance.

While the types of medical complications from cosmetic surgeries performed abroad overlap with those in the United States – primarily surgical site infections and wound dehiscence – studies note that patients traveling from developing countries carried home more unusual and resistant procedure-related infections requiring higher rates of hospitalization.[22] Cosmetic surgeries in Latin America were often associated with anaerobic bacteria, with a 2005 survey of North American infectious disease specialists finding that 6% of 425 respondents had encountered infectious complications including *Mycobacterium abscessus*, which has become increasingly common in patients seeking surgical cosmetic procedures abroad. Media reports of complications include septic shock from ruptured fraudulent breast implants, and necrotizing abscesses causing limb loss, organ failure, and death.[24]

Patients presenting with complications of cosmetic procedures performed abroad may be approached similarly to patients with complications of local procedures. The main difference in initial approach will be availability of information regarding the procedure. A detailed history inquiring about the procedure type and exam that identifies surgical wounds and approach may be required to figure out exactly what was done. Careful review of outside documentation, if available, should be performed. Familiarity with procedures that are commonly performed and their complications will aid in communicating with consulting surgeons.

Organ Transplant

Transplant tourism, a subset of medical tourism where a patient travels to another country to acquire an organ, makes up 10% of all solid organ transplants globally.[25] In 2010, 98 countries reported organ transplant services and performed about 100,000 transplant surgeries annually.[26] While a large number of transplants are performed annually in the US, more than three times as many patients remain on waiting lists. The huge discrepancy in available organ transplants and the time-limited nature of procedures push individuals to travel outside the country to obtain organ transplants, where payment for organ donation may be legal, screening may be limited, and risk of complications high. Furthermore, screening of donor organs is not widespread in all countries, and patients may acquire viral hepatitis, cytomegalovirus, or HIV from donor organs. In addition, organ donors or medical tourists may often become colonized with highly resistant microorganisms, including vancomycin-resistant staphylococci and MDR Enterobacteriaceae, including isolates that were found in India highly resistant to all beta-lactam antimicrobials including carbapenems, and which have since been detected in many countries.

Medical Tourists to the United States

There is a smaller percentage of individuals who travel to the United States to seek care. About 0.5% of all air travelers entering the United States annually – between 100,000 and 200,000 people – list health treatment as a reason for visiting, citing access to advanced medical care as their reason for traveling.[27] Some health facilities, such as the Mayo Clinic, actively market their services overseas, and specialize in providing high-quality medical care to foreigners who are willing to pay.

More commonly, urban clinicians can expect to see patients who have received a provisional diagnosis abroad and have traveled to the United States to seek care without a specific referral. While the ED management of such patients is usually straightforward once it is recognized that they have already received a workup, it can be surprisingly challenging to obtain that history. Asking for copies of any medical records can be helpful; many will be written in English or contain enough familiar language so as to be interpretable. Depending on the specific condition many of these patients will require admission, especially if they lack health insurance or access to primary and specialty care. Building a robust system of care that allows for direct outpatient referral combined with access to a financial counselor or social worker who can aid new immigrants in applying for assistance may allow outpatient management.

Vignette Conclusion

Once admitted, the patient was treated with ceftriaxone. Blood cultures were negative and stool cultures grew *Campylobacter*. He was treated with several days of IV antibiotics for presumed enteric fever and discharged once improved. He returned shortly thereafter with worsened pain. Blood cultures at admission grew *Salmonella paratyphi*. He was treated with several weeks of IV antibiotics and ultimately recovered.

Pro-Tips

- History is everything – the only way to recognize that someone has traveled, and therefore what they are at risk for, is to ask them. Even savvy patients may fail to recall important high-risk exposures unless you directly inquire about them. Share the history you get with your consultants (particularly radiologists) as it may influence interpretation of the clinical situation.

- Stay informed – international travelers will present with novel diseases with which we have limited first-hand experience. In order to make these diagnoses we need to stay up to date on both what's going on in the world and familiarize ourselves with classic presentations of unfamiliar conditions.

- Make no assumptions – it is impossible to tell by looking at someone where they might have been or what activities they engage in. Always err on the side of asking.

- Know the capabilities of your institution (and how to get help) – diagnosing diseases of international travelers may require testing that is not routinely available. Know where you can send tests and how long it will take to get them done. Some conditions, such as severe malaria, require rapid treatment with drugs that are not routinely available. Know where you can get those resources if needed.

References

1. Freedman DO, Weld LH, Kozarsky PE, Fisk T, Robins R, Von Sonnenburg F, Keystone JS, Pandey P, Cetron MS, GeoSentinel Surveillance Network. Spectrum of disease and relation to place of exposure among ill returned travelers. *N Engl J Med*. 2006;354(2):119–130.

2. Upadhyay DK, Sittig DF, Singh H. Ebola US Patient Zero: lessons on misdiagnosis and effective use of electronic health records. *Diagnosis*. 2014;1(4):283–287.

3. Wilson ME, Weld LH, Boggild A, Keystone JS, Kain KC, von Sonnenburg F, Schwartz E, GeoSentinel Surveillance Network. Fever in returned travelers: results from the GeoSentinel Surveillance Network. *Clin Infect Dis*. 2007;44(12):1560–1568.

4. Nilles EJ, Arguin PM. Imported malaria: an update. *Am J Emerg Med*. 2012;30(6):972–980.

5. World Health Organization, Special Programme for Research and Training in Tropical Diseases. *Dengue: Guidelines for Diagnosis, Treatment, Prevention and Control*. World Health Organization, 2009.

6. CDC. *Treatment of Malaria: Guidelines for Clinicians (United States)*. 2020. Available from: www.cdc.gov/malaria/resources/pdf/Malaria_Treatment_Guidelines.pdf.

7. Simkhada PP, Sharma A, van Teijlingen ER, Beanland RL. Factors influencing sexual behaviour between tourists and tourism employees: a systematic review. *Nepal J Epidemiol*. 2016;6(1):530.

8. Lu TS, Holmes A, Noone C, Flaherty GT. Sun, sea and sex: a review of the sex tourism literature. *Trop Dis, Travel Med Vacc.* 2020;6(1).

9. Braun DL, Kouyos RD, Balmer B, Grube C, Weber R, Günthard HF. Frequency and spectrum of unexpected clinical manifestations of primary HIV-1 infection. *Clin Infect Dis.* 2015;61(6):1013–1021.

10. Gupta S, Gupta M, Bhardwaj S, Chugh T. Current clinical patterns of typhoid fever: a prospective study. *J Trop Med Hygiene.* 1985;88(6):377–381.

11. Mogasale V, Desai SN, Mogasale VV, Park JK, Ochiai RL, Wierzba TF. Case fatality rate and length of hospital stay among patients with typhoid intestinal perforation in developing countries: a systematic literature review. *PLoS One.* 2014;9(4):e93784.

12. Jensenius M, Schlagenhauf P, Loutan L, Parola P, Schwartz E, Leder K, Freedman DO, GeoSentinel Surveillance Network. Acute and potentially life-threatening tropical diseases in western travelers – a GeoSentinel Multicenter Study, 1996–2011. *Am J Trop Med Hygiene.* 2013;88(2):397–404.

13. CDC. Extensively Drug-Resistant Typhoid Fever in Pakistan. 2019. Available from: wwwnc.cdc.gov/travel/notices/watch/xdr-typhoid-fever-pakistan.

14. CDC. Testing Guidance New Zika and Dengue Testing Guidance (Updated November 2019). 2019. Available from: www.cdc.gov/zika/hc-clinicians/testing-guidance.html.

15. Harvey K, Esposito DH, Han P, Kozarsky P, Freedman DO, Plier DA, Sotir MJ, Centers for Disease Control and Prevention. Surveillance for travel-related disease – GeoSentinel surveillance system, United States, 1997–2011. *MMWR Surveill Summ.* 2013;62(3):1–23.

16. Hill DR. Health problems in a large cohort of Americans traveling to developing countries. *J Travel Med.* 2000;7(5):259–266.

17. Siddique A, Akram K, Zaman K, Laston S, Salam A, Majumdar R, Zaman K, Fronczak N, Laston S. Why treatment centres failed to prevent cholera deaths among Rwandan refugees in Goma, Zaire. *Lancet.* 1995;345(8946):359–361.

18. Shane AL, Mody RK, Crump JA, Tarr PI, Steiner TS, Kotloff K, Langley JM, Wanke C, Warren CA, Cheng AC, Cantey J, Pickering LK. 2017 Infectious Diseases Society of America clinical practice guidelines for the diagnosis and management of infectious diarrhea. *Clin Infect Dis.* 2017;65(12):e45–e80.

19. de Bruyn G, Hahn S, Borwick A. Antibiotic treatment for travellers' diarrhoea. *Cochrane Database of Syst Rev.* 2000;2000(3):CD002242.

20. Kantele A, Lääveri T. Extended-spectrum beta-lactamase-producing strains among diarrhoeagenic *Escherichia coli* – prospective traveller study with literature review. *J Travel Med.* 2022;29(1):taab042.

21. Borders PB. Quick Facts About Medical Tourism 2022. Available from: www.patientsbeyondborders.com/media.

22. Pereira RT, Malone CM, Flaherty GT. Aesthetic journeys: a review of cosmetic surgery tourism. *J Travel Med.* 2018;25(1):tay042.

23. Gale J. *How Thailand Became a Global Gender-Change Destination.* Bloomberg. 2015.

24. Moore W. Delray Beach woman warns of dangers of medical tourism after suffering from complications. WPTV 5: NBC; 2019. Available from: www.wptv.com/news/local-news/investigations/delray-beach-woman-warns-of-dangers-of-medical-tourism-after-suffering-from-complications.

25. Adido TO. *Transplant Tourism: An International and National Law Model to Prohibit Travelling Abroad for Illegal Organ Transplants.* Nijhoff, 2018.

26. Stoney RJ, Kozarsky PE, Walker AT, Gaines JL. Population-based surveillance of medical tourism among US residents from 11 states and territories: findings from the Behavioral Risk Factor Surveillance System. *Infect Control Hosp Epidemiol.* 2022; 43(7):870–875.

27. Chambers A. Trends in US health travel services trade. United States International Trade Commission Executive Briefing on Trade. 2015.

HIV, AIDS, and Tuberculosis

Marc Phillip Kanter, Trevor Mark Janus, and Marimer Rivera-Nieves

Vignette

A 48-year-old man with no known past medical history presents to the Emergency Department (ED), brought in by ambulance, for one week of progressive cough and shortness of breath. The patient also reports progressive weakness, generalized malaise, and a self-diagnosed "right eye infection" during the interval period. The emergency medical service providers found him to be hypoxemic and applied a non-rebreather mask with high-flow oxygen prior to his arrival at the ED. At the time of presentation, he is mildly hypoxic, but speaking in full sentences and does not show signs of respiratory distress.

On exam, his mucous membranes are dry, his right eye has a scleral injection; "track marks," stigmata of IV drug use, are noted on his limbs bilaterally; and there is a poorly healing wound on his left calf. Bedside ultrasound reveals a B/B profile with right lung consolidation and grossly poor ejection fraction on echocardiogram. An electrocardiogram shows sinus tachycardia. A portable chest x-ray reveals cardiomegaly with pulmonary edema, although an underlying pulmonary mass cannot be ruled out. Diagnostic testing is significant for leukopenia, mild hyponatremia, slightly elevated troponin, brain natriuretic peptide of greater than 5000, and lactate dehydrogenase greater than two times the upper limit of normal. Influenza and coronavirus disease 2019 (COVID-19) tests and legionella antigen are all negative.

- What exam findings are suggestive of tuberculosis (TB)?
- How does the urban setting influence the intersection of human immunodeficiency virus (HIV) and TB?

Introduction

In the ED, patients present with diverse infectious diseases. Some diseases require a keen eye from the clinician to diagnose and prevent transmission and progression. HIV and TB are two conditions that are easily overlooked in the ED, yet are the two deadliest infectious diseases in the world. The HIV/AIDS epidemic has been a challenge to the United States health system since the 1980s and continues to represent major health and economic burden. TB cases in the US had been down trending in the 1950s but since 1985 cases began to rise in urban areas where large communities of immigrants are present. The HIV and TB pandemics are largely intertwined as TB is a major cause of death in HIV patients. Most cases in the US are concentrated in urban areas of low income. Individuals of color, those experiencing homelessness, those engaging in high-risk sexual behavior, and those with substance use disorder are the most likely to be affected. Advances in therapeutics as well as the development of screening modalities have made significant progress. The ED is the major point of contact for diagnosis and linkage to long-term care.

HIV/AIDS

Epidemiology

Acquired immunodeficiency syndrome (AIDS) was first discovered in the United States in 1981 shortly after clusters of *Pneumocystis carinii* pneumonia and Kaposi's sarcoma cases were reported in communities of men-who-have-sex-with-men (MSM). The causative agent, the human immunodeficiency virus, would later be discovered in 1983. Between 1981 and 1986 all US states, territories, and the District of Columbia implemented mandated reporting of HIV/AIDS cases to the Centers for Disease Control and Prevention (CDC). Shortly after the implementation of a reporting system, it was demonstrated that most cases of HIV and AIDS, both incidence and prevalence, were in major metropolitan areas. This trend has continued with >80% of cases reported in these environments.

The AIDS epidemic continues to be a national health challenge in the United States and a crisis in its impoverished urban communities. The CDC recognizes an infection rate of 1% as an epidemic and according to their analysis, high-risk urban environments have infection rates at more than double this at 2.1%. These rates are on par with those seen in impoverished nations such as Haiti and Ethiopia.[1] Further analysis of these areas reveals neighborhoods of even higher concentrations of those affected.

At the start of the HIV/AIDS epidemic in America, this disease mostly affected white MSM in urban areas of high populations defined as >500,000. While the patterns of disease burden continue to be concentrated in dense urban settings, the groups of people disproportionately affected have changed. While the disease initially predominantly affected white MSM, infection rates now disproportionately affect Black and Hispanic urban communities. While overall incidence rates have remained relatively stable since the 1990s, the rates among those who are most likely to be affected have changed dramatically. Of new AIDS diagnoses, 75% were among MSM in the early 1980s but had dropped to 47% by the mid-2000s. At this time the chance of infection based on race/ethnicity also changed, with Black patients eight times more likely to contract HIV/AIDS when compared to their White urban counterparts; Hispanics were found to be three times as likely.[2,3]

Factors that influence the transmission of HIV and AIDS, especially in urban settings of dense populations, are complex and tied to the very fabric of the cities themselves. Differences in these infection rates are likely multifactorial and include race/ethnicity, income, and level of education. Driving factors for the epidemic include injection drug use and rates of same-sex and heterosexual contact, which differ between cities and the neighborhoods within them. For instance, injection drug use rates have been shown to differ from city to city by up to differences of 12-fold in likelihood.

Overall socioeconomic status (SES) has been demonstrated as being a significant risk factor for infection, with homelessness being a strong predictor. For instance, data that have been collected and reported from the District of Columbia, a city geographically divided by wards, have demonstrated an HIV prevalence of 0.4% in ward 3, where the population is of higher SES and predominately White. Contrast this with the predominantly Black citizens of the city of low SES in wards 5, 6, 7, and 8 where their prevalence is as high as 3.1%. This can also be illustrated in New York City, which has an overall infection rate of 1.4% in contrast to higher rates in neighborhoods with lower SES. Harlem, as well as Highbridge Morrisania and Hunts Point-Mott Haven (both neighborhoods of the Bronx), have infection rates of 2.4–4.5%.[2]

The level of significance that SES has on infection rates and disease-related mortality and morbidity can be seen in New York City. In the predominately White and relatively high SES neighborhood of Chelsea, the prevalence of HIV is similar to those seen in the Bronx and Harlem, but the death rates due to AIDS and AIDS-related diseases are starkly lower.

Other factors that may lead to the epidemic include an assumed increase in prevalence rates as improvements are made in retroviral therapies and that early detection will result in longer life spans and more positive outcomes in those infected.

Strategy and Screening

The Department of Health and Human Services (HHS) has addressed many of the disparities in its National Strategic Plan for 2021–2025. Priority populations include MSM with an emphasis on Black, Latinx, and American Indian/Alaska Native men. Other priority populations include Black women, transgender women, young people ages 13–24, and intravenous drug users. The broad national goals include reducing overall new infection rates, increasing pre-exposure prophylaxis (PrEP) coverage, linkage to care, increasing overall knowledge of HIV, increasing viral suppression, decreasing stigma, and decreasing homelessness among those infected. Per their report, progress has been made in decreasing incidence and increasing viral suppression. Health insurance coverage has largely improved for HIV treatment and increased NIH funding has been implemented.[4]

HIV screening for all pregnant persons is a United States Preventative Service Task Force (USPSTF) grade A recommendation, as does a one-time screening for all-comers ages 15–65 in medical settings including EDs, where undiagnosed infection rates tend to be high. The CDC recommends linkage to primary care for treatment within 30 days of diagnosis.[5] Multiple studies in different US cities have demonstrated that patients in neighborhoods of lower SES are less likely to interface with traditional primary care providers and more likely to access care through safety-net medical systems.[6]

The United States Department of HHS has published the lofty but theoretically possible goal of reducing HIV incidence to zero in the US by 2030. On top of the traditional screenings done in EDs and other clinical settings, other high-impact tactics that focus on marginalized populations have had varied results. A review of 51 public health jurisdictions has shown contact tracing to be relatively ineffective. However, the Social Network Strategy, recently endorsed by the CDC, has shown promising results. This is where HIV-positive or high-risk individuals are asked to recruit those in their social network for testing in exchange for an incentive, although the full cost of this strategy has yet to be fully quantified.[7]

Cities and local governments have implemented different strategies to combat the AIDS epidemic with varying degrees of success. In New York, the Bronx Knows project has taken aim at increasing voluntary testing and increased availability to care and prevention strategies. Other cities, like the District of Columbia, have introduced needle exchange and condom distribution programs. By offering HIV testing in EDs, patients can be connected to early intervention and treatment, hopefully reducing transmission rates and complications of HIV.

The role of the emergency physician is now to recognize this disease as early as possible. A thorough history and physical exam to find any signs suggestive of immunosuppression is required. Recurring fever, night sweats, and extreme and unexplained fatigue can be signs of undiagnosed HIV/AIDS. Unfortunately, few exam findings are specific to early HIV infection. Most commonly these patients will present with symptoms of a common cold, such as fevers, chills, sore throat, lymphadenopathy, rash, diarrhea, or myalgias and malaise. Thrush, temporal wasting, and signs of any AIDS-defining illness can be seen in more advanced cases or patients who have been sexually active with an HIV-positive patient. Primary HIV infection mimics general viral illness but is often more severe. In primary HIV infection examination of the oropharynx, genitals, and lymph nodes may be helpful. Obviously, any patient presenting with an AIDS-defining illness such as Kaposi sarcoma with no prior diagnosis warrants testing and possibly admission. Considering the clinical presentation of the patient and their history we should identify those patients that may be at higher risk of infection and test them. High-risk sexual behavior, incarceration, and intravenous drug use should pique the clinician's suspicion for testing, as should unexplained leukopenia.

In the ED, patients may be offered HIV testing during their visit, which may assist in early diagnosis of disease and prevent further complications. Ideally, a rapid HIV test and a viral load can be ordered while in the ED; the idea behind both is that a patient may test negative in a rapid test but if they have an increasing viral load early diagnosis would be made, although this requires follow-up results after the visit. Once diagnosed, these patients require follow-up with the infectious disease for treatment. Patients with known HIV who have close follow-up will present to the ED and know their CD4 count, which is helpful in diagnosing and treating concomitant diseases they may present with. If a patient does not know their CD4 count, a complete blood count (CBC) may be of assistance in estimating it. The absolute lymphocyte count (ALC) has been found to have a reliable relationship with CD4 count, for which reason it may be used to estimate a patient's CD4 count. Studies state that an ALC of <1000 cells/mm^3 is predictive of a CD4 less than 200 cells/mm^3 and an ALC ≥2000 cells/mm^3 is predictive of a CD4 over 200 cells/mm.^{3} Using this estimation, a physician can better treat a patient with concomitant diseases in the ED.[8]

Therapy

Treatment options for HIV infection have improved significantly since its discovery in the 1980s. Triple combination highly active antiretroviral therapy (HAART) remains the standard of care and single-tablet formulations now exist. Lower pill burden and decreased side-effect profiles have led to an overall increase in medication adherence. However, without a definitive cure, infected patients still require life-long therapy. This can pose yet another barrier to urban dwellers, especially those of low SES. Early trials of HAART therapy boasted very promising results with over 70% of patients achieving virologic suppression. However, many of these trials were tested in Caucasian males, potentially limiting their external validity when applied to a great number of urban neighborhoods and settings. When similar trials were implemented in urban settings with low-SES populations, the chances of virologic suppression were much lower: just over half that seen in the Caucasian trials.

When a clinician diagnoses a patient with acute HIV in the ED it is important in the management of the patient to refer them to an HIV specialist to be started on HAART.

When managing this patient, it is important to give good counseling on abstinence, safe sex, and avoiding needle sharing if they are an intravenous drug user to help prevent transmission. HIV is a reportable disease, and it is important to track and test any contact with patients that might have been exposed. Patients with known HIV should be already on HAART, but many will be non-compliant and fail to follow-up, for which reason they will present with unknown CD4 counts. Patients with chronic HIV will present to ED for diverse infections secondary to opportunistic pathogens. Patients should be started on antibiotics, which will be guided by the CD4 count and the associated opportunistic infection suspected. Most common pathogens are mentioned in Table 7.1.

Well-powered cohort studies have demonstrated that being of Black or Hispanic race/ethnicity, female, uninsured, or insured by Medicaid were all risk factors for receiving suboptimal HIV care. In multiple studies, substance use, especially cocaine, has been identified as a major barrier to antiretroviral care. Substance abuse has also been linked to a decreased likelihood of having or maintaining a relationship with a primary care provider. Antiretroviral non-adherence rates have been shown to be lower in monolingual non-English speakers.[9] Another barrier unique to urban citizens of low SES, especially the undomiciled, is a psychiatric disease, which has been shown to be an independent risk factor for maintaining care.

Tuberculosis

Tuberculosis (TB) is thought to have originated over 150 million years ago. TB became an epidemic around the eighteenth to nineteenth centuries in Europe and North America. In 1890, Hermann Heinrich Robert Koch made a presentation to the Tenth International Medical Conference in Berlin in which he presented the structure of a tubercle bacillus giving tuberculosis its name.[10]

Mycobacterium tuberculosis is an acid-fast bacillus known for causing TB in humans. *M. tuberculosis* replicates in humans after bacteria gain access to the host through aerosolized respiratory secretions that make their way through the respiratory tract. Once in the

Table 7.1 Patients With HIV Are At Risk of Many Opportunistic Infections. This Table Lists the Most Common Opportunistic Infections Associated With Decreased CD4 Counts.

CD4 count	Associated opportunistic infections
<500	Oral candidiasis (thrush) Kaposi sarcoma
<200	*Pneumocystis* pneumonia (PJP) Progressive multifocal leukoencephalopathy John Cunningham (JC) virus Chronic *Cryptosporidium* diarrhea
<100	Cerebral toxoplasmosis Systemic histoplasmosis *Candida* esophagitis
<50	Cryptococcal meningitis Cytomegalovirus (CMV) retinitis *Mycobaterium avium* complex (MAC)

lungs, an inflammatory cascade begins. Macrophages in the lungs attempt to clear the body from bacteria by phagocytosis to destroy the pathogen. When macrophages are unable to destroy the bacteria, they will replicate logarithmically within the macrophages. *M. tuberculosis* has a long replication time as it is non-motile and cell division can take up to 24 hours, which is why immediate exposure will not yield positive results when testing.[11,12] When TB is activated, it may stay in the lungs and cause a local infection; primary or pulmonary TB; or it may travel through the lymph nodes to other areas of the body and cause extrapulmonary infections.[11] Many humans will get inoculated with the bacteria but will not present with the disease until years later, making latent TB the most common cause of TB-infected individuals in the world.[12]

Epidemiology of TB

TB is a common disease worldwide, affecting nearly one quarter of the world's population. In 2020, the CDC reported 7174 new cases of TB in the United States, a rate of 2.2 cases per 100,000 population. Most TB cases reported occur in persons born outside of the US, most commonly from Mexico, the Philippines, India, Vietnam, and China.[13] Over 50% of the active TB cases reported in the United States currently occur in foreign-born individuals, with the majority being the result of the reactivation of latent TB.[14,15] Anyone can get TB, but Asians, Hispanics or Latinos, non-Hispanic Blacks, or African Americans have been shown to be' at the highest risk. TB is more common in males of any age than females. Males accounted for over 60% of cases of TB in 2020.[16]

In 2020, 9 million people contracted TB around the world and 1.1 million of those were children. Approximately 2 million people die of TB each year in countries outside the United States.[13] A study performed in Zambia showed that the prevalence of TB was 3% higher in the urban setting than in rural areas, but there is a higher risk of death from TB in the rural setting due to patients being lost to follow-up.[17] A study in Denmark showed the incidence of TB in urban areas was twice as high than in rural areas.[15] Urban areas carry a higher risk of TB infection due to marginalization of the population such as homelessness, HIV epidemic, poor SES, lack of access to quality healthcare, and incarceration.[13,15] TB is a treatable disease if diagnosed, so it is important to monitor and treat it correctly. The CDC and the World Health Organization (WHO) invest in research every year to ensure proper surveillance of TB and treatment as it is a preventable and treatable disease.

TB in the United States

In 1892, TB became a reportable disease in the United States. New York City served as a model for the US Public Health Service, including public education, testing, and follow-up.[10] From 1953 to 1985, there was a decrease in reported tuberculosis cases in the United States, and cases were down 75%. In 1985, however, there was an increase in TB cases, the majority being detected in New York City. The sharp rise in cases was linked to the HIV epidemic. In the United States, the majority of cases are seen in urban cities due to immigration, low SES, and high population density. Studies have shown that the incidence in urban areas is twice as high as that in rural areas.[14,15] Since 1992, the incidence of TB in the United States has dropped every year and continues dropping worldwide.[13] While TB has decreased in incidence in the United States, it remains an important infection to diagnose and treat.

TB elimination would have widespread health benefits. The WHO created *The End TB Strategy* with the goal to eliminate TB worldwide by 2035. To achieve this goal, they are expanding care, strengthening prevention, and expanding research. To achieve elimination of TB, physicians must continue being aware of the disease to diagnose it in time and treat it. TB is a reportable disease by law and should be reported to the health department within 24 hours of diagnosis. Government funding exists to cover TB testing and treatment for patients with no insurance and many assistance programs exist for patients with insurance that may not be able to afford such medications. Many state health departments will continue the process of monitoring patients, evaluating their close contacts for the disease, and ensuring proper treatment.

Emergency department clinicians' involvement in the diagnosis and management of patients with suspected active TB begins with thorough screening. A focused review of systems and an assessment of risk factors by a primary provider will be key for initiating the proper workup and management for patients with TB. Clinicians in urban areas should maintain tuberculosis in their differentials when treating immigrants, HIV, the homeless, or the incarcerated with coughs, fevers, night sweats, and weight loss. Patients with TB may present to the ED with either a primary infection or, more commonly, reactivation of latent TB. In either event, a wide variety of symptoms are features of this disease. ED presentations include classic infection in previously undiagnosed TB, TB with atypical symptoms, and known TB history with incomplete or complete drug therapy. TB may present with infection to the lungs or extrapulmonary infections. In immunocompetent hosts, 85% of reported cases have only pulmonary involvement; by contrast, in immunocompromised hosts (like patients with HIV/AIDS), TB infection may present with pulmonary involvement (38%), extrapulmonary involvement (30%), and combined features (32%).[6]

TB most commonly affects the lungs as it is the first site the pathogen infects. If TB gets activated in the lungs it causes pulmonary TB. Patients with pulmonary TB will present with a constellation of systemic and pulmonary symptoms like fevers, chills, pleuritic chest pain, cough, and, on occasion, unilateral pleural effusion on chest x-ray. The initial cough of TB will be dry and as tissue damage progresses and tissue necrosis ensues, green sputum and hemoptysis will develop.[6] Physical exam findings are non-specific; rales and rhonchi may be present over areas of consolidation or decreased breath sounds in areas of effusion. When pulmonary TB is in the differential, a chest x-ray will help rule in the diagnosis. Over 70% of patients with TB will present with an abnormal x-ray. The classic x-ray finding is the Ghon complex, which is the caseating granuloma in the middle lung lobe which is only seen when calcified with ipsilateral mediastinal lymphadenopathy. To confirm the diagnosis, three sputum cultures should be collected in consecutive days. To collect sputum, patients should be in isolation and saline may be used to induce sputum production. Some countries rely solely on a positive smear to diagnose TB, but in the US there must be growth of the organism in a culture medium for patients to be considered infected.[8] Other presentations of pulmonary TB may not be due to primary infection but to reactivation or secondary TB. In these cases, patients may present the same as primary TB except x-ray findings most commonly will present cavitary lesions in the apices of the lung.

TB may spread through lymph nodes and the hematologic system causing infection in bones, the central nervous system, the heart, the gastrointestinal system, and more. Patients will present with fevers, chills, malaise, and symptoms specific to the site of infection. Patients with pulmonary miliary TB will present with a reticulonodular pattern with pulmonary opacities on chest x-ray of 2 mm or less.

Many patients will present with extrapulmonary TB. One of the most common presentations is lymphadenitis. Thirty-one percent of cases of extrapulmonary TB are due to TB infection of the lymph nodes (ralias media). Generally, the adenopathy will present unilateral and non-tender with matted nodes on the exam. Patients will commonly present with adenopathy to the cervical, mediastinal, and axillary nodes. Scrofula, cervical chain lymphadenopathy, sometimes can extend through the skin and form a fistula. Extrapulmonary TB may be infectious when present in the oral cavity or in an open skin lesion.[15]

Management and Disposition

When treating a patient with high suspicion of TB, the patient should be placed in a negative-pressure room and airborne isolation precautions should be taken when treating the patient. Physicians and nurses caring for the patient should always wear a properly fit-tested N95 mask to prevent the risk of infection. TB is a treatable infection that can be eradicated if patients are diagnosed early and treated correctly. Many patients seen in the ED will have barriers to care (including homelessness, low income, and poor access to follow-up care), and it is the job of the ED physician to diagnose these patients correctly and decrease the spread. Stable patients may be admitted for further workup of pulmonary or extrapulmonary TB. Treatment can be initiated after a positive culture or high suspicion from imaging and thorough history. Patients with severe infections like miliary TB or meningitis should be started on a medical regimen immediately.

Patients diagnosed with TB should be started on the four-drug regimen known as RIPE, which stands for rifampin, isoniazid, pyrazinamide, and ethambutol. Treatment should begin as soon as a diagnosis is made, and the patient should remain on it for at least 6–9 months with continuous cultures to monitor treatment efficacy.

Upon reassessment of cultures, if no TB is found after 2 months then a two-drug regimen, rifampin and ethambutol, may be continued for the remaining 4–7 months.

Many patients will be infected with TB and never present with symptoms; this is called latent TB. Patients with latent TB may be treated with isoniazid alone for 9 months with added pyridoxine. INH alone is appropriate for recent asymptomatic skin test conversion in any person in close contact with an actively infected patient and anergic patients with known tuberculosis contact. Special consideration is taken when treating pregnant patients with TB. For active TB in a pregnant woman, the regimen should consist of 9 months of INH, rifampin, and ethambutol. The current literature does not recommend discontinuation of breastfeeding during this period. Also, pyridoxine supplementation is recommended for all pregnant and lactating women.

Infectious disease consult should be placed for proper medication management. Multidrug-resistant TB (MDRT) is a growing issue and should be monitored by a specialist. Some strains of M. tuberculosis are resistant to rifampin and ethambutol. These patients should be evaluated by specialists for proper treatment.

It is very important to ensure good follow-up for all TB patients as medication non-compliance is one of the major reasons MDRT exists.[6] Non-adherence to medication may be due to poor SES, poor support, inability to obtain medications, and more, for which reason the CDC and the WHO continue to work with health departments to warrant funding for medication availability and monitoring of these patients. Most city, state, and regional health departments in the United States have a TB program that maintains a patient registry but also provides support for testing, treatment, and follow-up. In addition to facility resources, ED clinicians should utilize local health department resources for any cases that raise diagnostic, treatment, ethical, or medico-legal concerns. To guarantee the eradication of this infection, it is important to ensure proper treatment.

Vignette Conclusion

Given the findings, the patient is offered HIV testing, which is found to be positive and confirmed through antibody testing. Infectious disease is consulted, and the patient is admitted to the medical intensive care unit. The viral load is found to be over 100,000 copies per mL. CD4 count is found to be less than 100.

HIV is an epidemic of great significance in the United States. It represents a major source of morbidity and mortality for those infected, continues to be a disease of stigma, and is a substantial burden on the American healthcare system. While all areas of the US are affected, urban communities bear the brunt of this burden. US cities were the first, and are likely to be the last, battlegrounds in the fight against this disease. HIV/AIDS has also caused an increase in the incidence of TB, making both of these illnesses two of the major infectious diseases causing death in the world. The emergency medicine clinician must consider both of these infections in an urban setting and test for them appropriately. Accurate diagnosis and rapid therapy can improve patient outcomes and reduce the spread of these diseases.

Pro-Tips

- HIV and TB are reportable diseases to the CDC. Know your local, county, and state Department of Health reporting regulations.
- HIV can be a silent disease process in its early stages and early diagnosis imparts better outcomes; the emergency clinician should maintain constant vigilance.
- Early detection of both diseases is very important. Both TB and HIV are treatable, and early detection and treatment reduces transmission and downstream morbidity.
- Patients with apparent viral syndromes may have HIV or TB. A thorough history and physical are crucial to identify factors that help to make these diagnoses.
- TB may present with pulmonary symptoms and/or non-pulmonary symptoms; these patients need to be isolated, and infectious diseases must be consulted for further evaluation and management.
- Risk factors include low SES (especially homelessness), injection drug use, high-risk sexual behavior, and infection with other sexually transmitted infections.

References

1. Denning P, DiNenno E. Communities in crisis: is there a generalized HIV epidemic in impoverished urban areas of the United States? Presented at XVIII International AIDS Conference (AIDS 2010), Vienna, Austria. 2010.

2. Nunn A, Yolken A, Cutler B, Trooskin S, Wilson P, Little S, Mayer K. Geography should not be destiny: focusing HIV/AIDS implementation research and programs on microepidemics in US neighborhoods. *Am J Public Health.* 2014;104:775–780. doi.org/10.2105/AJPH.2013.301864

3. Hall HI, Espinoza L, Benbow N, Hu YW, for the Urban Areas HIV Surveillance Workgroup. Epidemiology of HIV infection in large urban areas in the United States.

PLoS One. 2010;5(9):e12756. https://doi .org/10.1371/journal.pone.0012756

4. Department of Health and Human Services. *National Strategic Plan. A Roadmap to End the Epidemic for the United States 2021–2025.* Department of Health and Human Services, 2021.

5. Leider J, Fettig J, Calderon Y. Engaging HIV-positive individuals in specialized care from an urban emergency department. *AIDS Patient Care STDS.* 2011;25(2):89–93. doi:10.1089/apc.2010.0205

6. Reliasmedia.com. *Tuberculosis: A Primer for the Emergency Physician* [online]. 2022. Available at: www.reliasmedia.com/art icles/100438-tuberculosis-a-primer-for-the-emergency-physician (accessed January 28, 2022).

7. Skaathun B, Pho MT, Pollack HA, Friedman SR, McNulty MC, Friedman EE, Schmitt J, Pitrak D, Schneider JA. Comparison of effectiveness and cost for different HIV screening strategies implemented at large urban medical centre in the United States. *J Int AIDS Soc.* 2020;23 (10):e25554. doi:10.1002/jia2.25554. PMID: 33119195; PMCID: PMC7594703.

8. Shapiro NI, Karras DJ, Leech SH, Heilpern KL. Absolute lymphocyte count as a predictor of CD4 count. *Ann Emerg Med.* 1998;32(3 Pt 1):323–328. doi:10.1016/ s0196-0644(98)70008-3. PMID: 9737494.

9. Hussein M, Diez Roux AV, Field RI. Neighborhood socioeconomic status and primary health care: usual points of access and temporal trends in a major US urban area. *J Urban Health.* 2016;93(6):1027–1045. doi:10.1007/

s11524-016-0085-2. Erratum in: *J Urban Health.* 2016;93(6):1046. PMID: 27718048; PMCID: PMC5126022.

10. Daniel TM. The history of tuberculosis. *Respir Med.* 2006;100(11):1862–1870. https://doi.org/10.1016/j.rmed.2006.08.006.

11. Maison DP. Tuberculosis pathophysiology and anti-VEGF intervention. *J Clin Tuberc Other Mycobact Dis.* 2022;27:100300. https:// doi.org/10.1016/j.jctube.2022.100300

12. Center of Disease Control and Prevention. Transmission and pathogenesis of tuberculosis. Retrieved January 1, 2022, from www.cdc.gov/tb/education/corecurr/ pdf/chapter2.pdf

13. Sia IG, Wieland ML. Current concepts in the management of tuberculosis. *Mayo Clin Proc.* 2011:86(4):348–361.

14. Adigun R, Singh R. Tuberculosis. StatPearls. 2022. Available from www .ncbi.nlm.nih.gov/books/NBK441916/

15. Oren E, Winston CA, Pratt R, Robison VA, Narita M. Epidemiology of urban tuberculosis in the United States, 2000– 2007. *Am J Public Health.* 2011;101 (7):1256–1263. doi:10.2105/ AJPH.2010.300030

16. Centers for Disease Control and Prevention. Tuberculosis. 2022. Retrieved from www.cdc.gov/tb/default.htm

17. Mutembo S, Mutanga JN, Musokotwane K, Kanene C, Dobbin K, Yao X, Li C, Marconi VC, Whalen CC. Urban–rural disparities in treatment outcomes among recurrent TB cases in Southern Province, Zambia. *BMC Infect Dis.* 2019;19(1):1087. doi:10.1186/s12879-019-4709-5

Further Reading

1. Trepka MJ, Fennie KP, Sheehan DM, Lutfi K, Maddox L, Lieb S. Late HIV diagnosis: differences by rural/urban residence, Florida, 2007–2011. *AIDS Patient Care STDS.* 2014;28(4):188–197. doi:10.1089/apc.2013.0362

2. Sarno EL, Bettin E, Jozsa K, Newcomb ME. Sexual health of rural and urban young male couples in the United States: differences in HIV testing, pre-exposure prophylaxis use,

and condom use. *AIDS Behav.* 2021;25 (1):191–202. doi.org/10.1007/s10461-020- 02961-8.

3. El-Sadr WM, Mayer KH, Hodder SL. AIDS in America – Forgotten but not gone. *New Engl J Med.* 2010;362(11):967–970. doi:10.1056/NEJMp1000069

4. Spaulding AC, MacGowan RJ, Copeland B, Shrestha RK, Bowden CJ, Kim MJ, Margolis A, Mustaafaa G, Reid LC,

Heilpern KL, Shah BB. Costs of rapid HIV screening in an urban emergency department and a nearby county jail in the southeastern United States. *PLoS One.* 2015;10(6):e0128408. https://doi.org/10.1371/journal.pone.0128408

5. Reif S, Golin CE, Smith SR. Barriers to accessing HIV/AIDS care in North Carolina: rural and urban differences. *AIDS Care.* 2005;17(5):558–565. doi:10.1080/09540120412331319750

6. Haukoos JS, Mehta SD, Harvey L, Calderon Y, Rothman RE. Research priorities for human immunodeficiency virus and sexually transmitted infections surveillance, screening, and intervention in emergency departments: consensus-based recommendations. *Acad Emerg Med.* 2009;16(11):1096–1102. doi:10.1111/j.1553-2712.2009.00546.x. PMID: 20053228; PMCID: PMC4733316.

7. Blanchard E, Klibanov OM, Axelrod P, Palermo B, Samuel R. Virologic success in an urban HIV clinic: outcome at 12 months in patients who were HAART naïve. *HIV Clin Trials.* 2008;9(3):186–191. doi:10.1310/hct0903-186. PMID: 18547905.

8. Peto HM, Pratt RH, Harrington TA, LoBue PA, Armstrong LR. Epidemiology of extrapulmonary tuberculosis in the United States, 1993–2006. *Clin Infect Dis.* 2009;49(9):1350–1357. doi:10.1086/605559. PMID: 19793000.

9. Wang E, Sohoni A. Tuberculosis: a primer for the emergency physician. *Emerg Med Rep.* 2006. www.reliasmedia.com/articles/100438-tuberculosis-a-primer-for-the-emergency-physician (accessed January 29, 2022).

Chapter

8

Asthma

Claudia Sofia Simich and Michael P. Jones

Vignette 1

A 12-year-old boy is brought to the emergency department (ED) by his grandmother with shortness of breath for 2 days. There was a recent building fire in the adjacent building and his grandmother reports that the smell of smoke has been lingering. She notes that he often comes to the ED during the spring and summer months and has to avoid dogs and neighbors who smoke cigarettes in the apartment complex. Of note, it has been extremely hot and humid and the family has been trying to reduce their use of air conditioning due to the increased cost of electricity.

   Vitals: HR: 124, BP: 108/60, RR: 28, Sat: 92% on room air

   The exam is significant for labored breathing, decreased breath sounds with diffuse wheezing. The ED physician initiates treatment.

- What factors are unique to this child's asthma care in an urban setting?
- What socioeconomic factors play an important role in long-term morbidity and mortality?

Vignette 2

Carl is a 55-year-old male who is brought to the ED. Police officers are at his bedside attempting to take a statement but he is very short of breath and states he is an asthmatic. Carl was walking through the park with a friend when he witnessed an individual push a school kid to the ground and run off with his backpack. The child was unharmed and surrounded by Good Samaritans who contacted the police. Carl chased after the perpetrator and was able to tackle him and retrieve the backpack. Police arrived shortly after and arrested the perpetrator and also arranged for immediate transport to the hospital. He notes that when he runs, he needs his inhaler, which he did not have at the time.

   Vitals: HR: 116, BP: 156/110, RR: 26, Sat: 90% on room air

   The exam is significant for diaphoresis, several abrasions to his arms and legs, and diffuse bilateral wheezing. The ED physician initiates treatment.

- Are there special factors in this patient's care in an urban setting? What other issues could contribute to this patient's difficulty breathing?
- How does access to asthma care inhibit effective home management and care?

Introduction

Asthma is one of the leading respiratory complaints presenting to EDs and a prevalent cause of hospitalizations. Urban environments present special issues related to the pathophysiology, underlying causative conditions, management, and long-term outcomes. Environmental pollutants and traffic-related pollution are two important factors affecting urban asthmatics. There are also significant socioeconomic and numerous social determinants of health that impact urban environments in the management of asthma. These conditions affect prevalence, morbidity, and mortality, so a holistic approach to management and treatment is crucial for the patient's outcome. Understanding these differences can help identify opportunities for improved management on the individual and population basis.

Pathophysiology

Asthma is classified as a chronic inflammatory and obstructive pulmonary disease. It is characterized by a limitation of airflow secondary to airway inflammation, bronchial hypersensitivity, and a reversible airflow obstruction.[1] Patients with asthma have a known hyperresponsiveness to allergenic antigens and non-allergenic stimuli that cause bronchoconstriction leading to airflow obstruction. The longer asthma goes untreated, the more airway resistance increases, leading to air trapping and eventual respiratory fatigue and ventilatory failure.

Precipitants of asthma exacerbations include pollen, house dust, mold, pests, cats, dogs, viral infections, cleaners and disinfectants, tobacco, smoke, changes in humidity, changes in temperatures, and medications, among others. Antigens can activate mast cells and trigger inflammatory mediators and metabolic products that cause vasoconstriction, vascular congestion, and edema formation.[2] The combination of bronchial wall edema, inflammation, thickened mucous production, and airway smooth muscle contraction and hypertrophy lead to a narrowing in the diameter of the airway causing airflow obstruction, and subsequent respiratory distress and failure. The overwhelming majority of triggers are environmental or viral, but many are non-specific or unidentifiable. Environmental factors are particularly significant because they have been associated with asthma exacerbations and asthma development. Outdoor air pollutants that impact asthma are particulate matter (PM), ground-level ozone (O_3), nitrogen dioxide (NO_2), and sulfur dioxide (SO_2).[3] Other outdoor allergens include grass, weed pollen, spores, and trees that tend to vary in concentrations seasonally.

Clinical Features

Classic symptoms of asthma include shortness of breath, wheezing, chest tightness, and cough. Symptoms can present acutely, within minutes after an exposure to a trigger, or gradually over days. Nocturnal worsening is common. Chronic asthmatics may present with vague symptoms like trouble sleeping, feelings of tiredness, and decreased activity. Physical exam findings include wheezing, prolonged expiratory phase, and episodic cough. Severe asthma exacerbations can present in a tripod position gasping for air with tachypnea, tachycardia, hypoxia, diaphoresis, increased work of breathing, inability to speak in complete sentences, use of accessory muscles of respiratory, and paradoxical movement of the diaphragm and abdomen during inspiration. Patients typically have decreased inspiratory to expiratory ratios, pulsus paradoxus, and mucus plugging.[2] Severe airflow obstruction and impending respiratory muscle fatigue cause hypercapnia. Signs of hypercapnia include lethargy, altered mental status, tremors, plethora, unconsciousness, and apnea. Intubation should be done prior to or immediately upon development of these symptoms.

It is important to note that the degree of wheezing does not correlate with the severity of air flow obstruction; a quiet chest with poor air movement can be present with severe obstructions and impending respiratory failure. Equally important to clarify is the adage that "not everything that wheezes is asthma." While asthma can initially be developed at any age group, there are other causes of wheezing like congestive heart failure (CHF), chronic obstructive pulmonary disease (COPD), cardiomyopathy, or lung cancer.[1] In children, it is especially important to evaluate for foreign body aspiration.

Epidemiology

Asthma is a common illness that affects up to 7.8% of the entire population in the United States. According to the Centers of Disease Control and Prevention (CDC), over 25 million adults and children suffer from asthma in the United States as of 2020. This number accounts for patients who have been formally diagnosed; many more go undiagnosed. Of those who identify as having asthma, 41% had an asthma attack in 2020, 18% visited an ED, and 7.3% required a hospital inpatient stay.[4] There has been a 43% increase in asthma incidence since 1990 to 2018 in the United States.[5]

In the United States, asthma is more common in young adults (ages 20–39) and teenagers than the elderly (greater than 65). It is more common in females than males at a ratio of 3:2. The asthma ED visits rate (per 10,000 population) is significantly higher among children (88.1) than among adults (42.1) and among women (50.4) than among men (31.1). Also, ED visit rates significantly reduce with increasing age: 62.7 among adults aged 18–34 years, 36.9 among adults aged 35–64 years, and 18.2 among adults aged 65 years and over.[4]

The groups with the highest prevalence of asthma in the United States are American Indians and Alaskan Natives followed closely by Black non-Hispanics.[4] Asthma is more prevalent in people living below the poverty threshold, making up approximately 16% (roughly 4 million) of the total asthma cases in the United States.[4] Asthma occurs more frequently in urban environments than in rural areas and this difference correlates with environmental risk exposure, healthcare access, and a patient's socioeconomic environment.

The World Health Organization reports that an estimate 262 million people suffered from asthma in 2019 and caused 455,000 deaths.[6] Asthma is one of the most common non-communicable diseases in the world, although it has a low mortality globally. The prevalence of asthma is higher in developed western countries; the prevalence of asthma in developed western countries is around 10% while it is ≤1% in developing countries.[7] Urbanization has a direct and synergistic correlation with the prevalence of asthma. North America has the highest prevalence of asthma (10,399.3 per 100,000) and East Asia has the lowest (2025.5 per 100,000) as per the Global Burden of Disease Report in 2019.[8] Although the incidence of asthma is lower in populations living in underdeveloped and eastern nations, hospital admissions (commonly used as an indicator of asthma care and control) vary greatly among countries due to a variety of factors affecting admissions.[9] There has been an overall reduction in hospital admission since 1990 in several countries, but admissions vary depending on accessibility and affordability to healthcare. Therefore, the utility of hospital admissions rates in understanding the global burden of asthma is very limited.[10]

Morbidity and Mortality

Chronic respiratory illness (asthma, COPD, emphysema, interstitial lung disease) was the third most common cause of death in the United States in both males and females in 2019.[9] They account for a total of 7.64% of total deaths in the United States in 2019, which is 68.6

deaths per 100,000. In 1990, chronic respiratory illness accounted for 41.84 deaths per 100,000 or 4.98% of total deaths.[9]

The CDC reports asthma mortality at a rate of 1.26 per 100,000 in 2020 when compared to the rate of 1.9 per 100,000 in 1990.[4] Asthma currently accounts for 4145 annual deaths in the United States. Despite these positive downward trends, mortality varies greatly among age, gender, and race. Adults over 65 years have the highest mortality rate at 30.7, while children under 18 years old have a mortality rate <5%. Females account for 60% of asthma mortality while males account for the other 40%. Black non-Hispanics have the highest mortality rate in both adults and children, accounting for 28.7% of mortality cases among adults and 58.3% of cases among children in 2020.[9] Non-white Hispanics have the lowest deaths per 100,000 cases among all races in both children and adults.

Although mortality has decreased in the United States, the morbidity of asthma has been increasing since 1990. According to the Global Burden of Disease Report in 2019, there were over 7 million years of healthy life lived with disability (YLD) due to chronic respiratory illness in the United States compared to 4 million in 1990.[9] Specifically, asthma caused 396 per 100,000 years of YLD in 2019 (a total of 1.3 million YDLs), compared to 357 per 100,000 in 1990 (a total of 90,000 YDLs).[9] Disability adjusted life years (DALY) measure the combined years of life due to premature mortality and years of life lost due to disability; one DALY represents the loss of the equivalent of one year of health. Asthma was ranked #19 in 2019 with a loss of 432 DALYs per 100,000 (a total of 1.4 million DALYs), when compared to 415 DALYs per 100,000 in 1990 (a total of 1.05 million DALYs).[9] In children below 15 years of age, asthma is the #1 cause of loss of DALYs and YLDs.

According to the United States Environmental Protection Agency (EPA) in 2013, the approximate financial burden of asthma in the United States is around $56 billion.[10] An estimated $50.1 billion is spent directly on hospital stays and the other $5.9 billion is from sickness, death, wages lost or missed school/workdays. According to a study that evaluated the economic burden of asthma in the US, the approximate cost of asthma per person in $3266 per year in 2013, with an increase of $315 for those living below the poverty line ($3581).[11] Pulmonary disease is the second leading cause of disability in America and asthma specifically ranks within the top 10 prevalent conditions that cause limitation to activity.

Environmental Factors

Asthma exacerbation and management are closely linked to both indoor and outdoor environments. Indoor air can contain pollutants such as secondhand smoke, ozone, nitrogen dioxide, and particulate matter.[12] Indoor ozone levels are dependent on outdoor ozone levels, which in the US are closely monitored by the EPA, but levels vary depending on the season (they tend to be higher in warm seasons). Nitrogen dioxide is a gas that is produced in high-temperature combustion; for example, with the use of gas stoves, furnaces, or fireplaces. Particulate matter is made of solid and liquid particles that are suspended in the air. They are obtained from an assortment of sources such as pollen, spores, plants, animal debris, bacteria, dust, sea salt, combustion from factories, motor vehicles, power plants, smoke, cooking exhaust, etc.[13] Indoor air also contains cleaning products, pet dander, dust mites, molds, cockroach allergens, and other rodent allergens.

Indoor ozone's effect on asthma has not been well studied, but it has been proven that secondhand smoke and particulate matter are linked to asthma morbidity.[13] Studies have had inconsistent results in demonstrating the association of nitrogen dioxide and asthma.

Some have demonstrated an increase in wheezing, chest tightness, breathlessness, and daytime asthma,[14] while others have found no association between nitrogen dioxide and respiratory symptoms.[13] Studies have shown that particulate matter concentration does increase respiratory symptoms, increase use of rescue medication, and decreases lung function.[15]

Other important indoor environmental allergens are dust mites, cockroach allergens, and rat allergens. Dust mite exposure is also associated with greater medication use, poorer lung function, and increase in asthma symptoms.[16] Cockroach allergens have been associated with poorer asthma care and increase in healthcare utilization. Inner-city children have a higher sensitization rate to cockroaches (~30–40%) than suburban children (~21%)[17] and most inner-city homes have detectable cockroach allergen levels.[18] Lastly, mice and rats are also common in urban areas. Mice and rats produce a urinary allergen that can easily become airborne and has long been known to cause occupational asthma. Mice and rats can be found in virtually all urban homes (~85–90%),[19] especially those with poor maintenance and multifamily homes. One multicenter study showed that children sensitized to rats had higher asthma hospitalization and more emergency medical visits than those not sensitized, and that inner-city children had a 21% sensitization.[20]

Outdoor air pollutants include ozone, carbon monoxide, particulate matter, nitrogen dioxide, and sulfur dioxide. Other outdoor environmental allergens that affect asthma include weeds, grass, trees, and molds. As stated previously, particulate matter increases hospitalization rates, exacerbations, and a decline in lung function in asthmatic, and nitrogen oxide increases airway inflammation. Sulfur dioxide is a gas that is released with the combustion of coal, oil, during energy production and other industrial processes. Increased levels of sulfur dioxide increase bronchoconstriction and enhance the response to inhaled allergens.[3]

Ozone at the ground level is a harmful air pollutant, and it increases in the summertime; therefore, it is nicknamed "summertime smog."[21] Ground-level ozone levels increase with vehicular traffic, power plants, and industrial operations. Higher levels of ozone have been shown to cause coughing, difficulty breathing, inflammation to the airway, asthma exacerbations, increase frequency of asthma attacks, reduce lung function, and increase the use of rescue medication.[22] The United States EPA tracks ground-level ozone daily and found higher levels of ground-level ozone near urban centers when compared to rural areas.[3]

The CDC conducted an air quality comparative study from 2008 to 2012 between rural and urban zones in the United States. Three patterns for air quality were used and all three measures suggested an improvement in air quality as zones become more rural.[23] The study showed that nitrogen oxides (the combination of nitrogen oxide and nitrogen dioxides), carbon monoxide, sulfur dioxides, ground-level ozone, and particulate matters were more concentrated in urban areas and that rural counties experienced fewer unhealthy air quality days than large urban counties. While studies have shown that the prevalence of asthma is similar in urban (7.1%) and rural settings (5.7%),[24] it is important to note the health disparities income, housing, transpiration, health coverage, food security, etc. have on urban patients.

Transportation and Urbanization

Traffic-related airborne pollution (TRAP) is a combination of combustion and non-combustion sources, such as road dust, brake wear, and tire wear.[3] Chronic exposure to traffic-related pollution impairs lung function in children even when experienced at low levels, and can significantly decrease their lung function.[22] Epidemiological studies have shown that TRAP has caused an increase in respiratory symptoms, changes in lung function, and increases in healthcare use. Similar studies have also demonstrated a clear and consistent relationship between TRAP and childhood asthma.[25]

According to the US Department of Transportation, many major US cities (particularly those with higher densities of cars, commercial shipping, and public transportation vehicles) have increased TRAP levels compared to rural settings.[26] Interestingly, while this increase is expected in large urban centers, the TRAP has also increased in urban areas (which includes the city itself and the surrounding areas).

Unsurprisingly, both the EPA and American Lung Association report higher levels of TRAP in major cities. While industrial airborne pollution has been decreasing over the years in most industrial nations, TRAP has been increasing. Increased urbanization goes hand in hand with TRAP. Both TRAP and industrial airborne pollution have been shown to contribute to asthma exacerbations.[3] The prevalence of asthma has increased over years, as have urbanization rates and TRAP; people living in urban areas tend to be more affected by this than people living in rural areas.[27]

Walkability, transit exposure, and traffic exposure are all important health disparities that increase with time spent outside. A study in Orange County, California in 2013 on low-income residence and subsidized housing showed that low-income residents lived in higher transit-accessible areas, with a higher likelihood of traffic exposure, and more walkable areas.[28] Transportation, walkability, and airborne pollution are all increased in urban areas, and their detrimental effects on asthma have been demonstrated.

Social Determinants of Health

The World Health Organization defines Social Determinants of Health (SDoH) as "non-medical factors that influence health outcomes. They are the conditions in which people are born, grow, work, live and age, and the wider set of forces and systems shaping the conditions of daily life."[29] The United States Department of Health and Healthy People 2030 divides the SDoH into five categories: neighborhood and physical environment, economic stability, education access and quality, healthcare access and quality, and social and community context. Economic stability greatly affects urban asthma. It is important to consider employment, income, expenses, debt, childcare coverage/cost, insurance status, and medical bills when contemplating treatment plans and possible discharges for asthma exacerbations. Low income has been shown to be associated with increased asthma exacerbations, hospitalization, incidence, and intensive care unit admissions despite race, education, or medication administration.[30] According to the United Stated Census Bureau, African Americans and Hispanics make up the majority of people living in poverty (the census did not specify American Indians or Alaskan Natives).[31]

While income makes up a part of economic stability it is not the only aspect that gives stability. According to the Urban Institute, informal employment is higher among immigrants who tend to live in urban areas.[32] Access to affordable child care, housing security, availability of paid sick days, debts, insurance status, and medical bills all contribute to a family's economic stability. The prevalence in asthma among those in the lowest economic bracket is multifactorial seeing as low-income households have less access to health care, less access to healthy food options, increased exposure to industrial pollution and TRAP, and poorer housing conditions.[33]

Access to quality education can also affect asthmatic patients. Low-quality education and educational inequities lead to limited health literacy. A study in 2019 showed the effects of low health literacy include "poor nutrition knowledge and behaviors, higher obesity rates, more medication errors, more emergency department use, and poor asthma knowledge, behavior, and outcomes."[34] Patients with lower educational levels have been shown to have a higher risk of developing asthma and an exacerbation after adjusting for sex, age, smoking and occupational exposures,[35] while other studies suggest access to proper treatment and a pulmonologist can make up for educational inequities.[36] Educational inequities continue to drive income inequities, which combined have a synergistic and negative effect on health literacy, asthma care, asthma control, ED visits, and overall quality of life.[36]

The social and community category of SDoH is broad, and includes interpersonal relations with family, friends, co-workers and members of the community, stress levels, safety in a neighborhood, discrimination, neglect, and racism. Evidence exists that these factors affect asthma. The mechanism as to how neighborhood violence increases asthma is not clear, but studies have shown that violence increases days of symptoms of an asthma exacerbation, suggesting heightened levels of cortisol and inflammatory markers as a possible culprit.[37] Other studies suggest that increased levels of stress associated with neighborhood violence are often also associated to risk factors like "poverty, smoking, second hand smoke, pollutants, limited access to healthcare or medications, reduced adherence to controller medication, unhealthy diet, and obesity" that combined worsen asthma control and morbidity.[38] Violence and stress do not just affect those who already have asthma; pregnant mothers with prenatal exposure to violent neighborhoods and stress have an increased risk of having children who wheeze at 2 years old[39] (even after accounting for cockroach allergen, pollutants and other confounders). Physical or sexual abuse also has been demonstrated to be associated with increased healthcare utilization for asthma exacerbation and increase use of asthma medications.[40]

Systemic racism has been demonstrated to have negative effects on health and causes an increase in health disparities. A study done in University of California San Francisco showed that participants who had not experienced racial discrimination in their care were twice as likely to have controlled asthma (37%) when compared to those who said they did experience racism (21%).[41] Although asthma is multifactorial and there are genetic and environmental predispositions, it is evident that racism affects housing opportunities, economic stability, educational opportunities, and access to healthcare. This combination causes higher disease prevalence, increased burden of disease, and diminished quality of life.

Food insecurity and access to healthy foods is another important social determinant of health. Poor diet is associated with inappropriate nutrition, increase in body mass index (BMI), and obesity. In turn, obesity is associated with multiple diseases like hypertension, coronary artery disease, hyperlipidemia, and diabetes that negatively affect asthma and its mortality. Healthier foods and diets rich in fruits and vegetables have been associated with diminished asthma symptoms and improvement in lung function.[42] Healthier foods are often more expensive and because the majority of the population living in poverty in the United States identify as African American and Hispanic, this noticeably creates racial inequities in obtaining optimal nutrition and diet quality. Healthier diets, diminished BMI, and increase in fruit and vegetable diets improve asthma symptoms and mortality.[43]

Access to healthcare is an important SDoH, and incorporates not only having quality access to healthcare but that the healthcare provided is in a timely, culturally respectful, and linguistically appropriate manner. While urban doctor-to-patient ratios are higher (53.3 doctors per 100,000 people) than rural doctor to patient ratios (39.8 doctors per 1000,000 people),[44] asthmatic patients in urban areas tend to have less access to doctors generally and to pulmonologists specifically. Many patients use the ED to obtain prescriptions for their rescue inhalers and their preventive regimens.

Segregation in neighborhoods can have an effect on pharmacies that tend to have inadequate medication supplies and hospitals that have limited resources, poor staffing ratios, overcrowding, and outdated medical equipment.[45] Specifically, asthmatic patients who lack health insurance, lack access to primary care, lack access to specialized care or lack access to their medications have higher ED utilization, increased school and work absence, numerous episodes of uncontrolled asthma, and overall worsening in their asthma care.

Treatment and Management

Treatment and management for asthma in urban centers largely mirrors the standard management – bronchodilators, inhaled and systemic corticosteroids, supplemental oxygen, and standard inpatient therapeutics. The complexity related to urban management relates to the unique socioeconomic and societal factors that may play a role in healthcare access and delivery.

Some of the important patient-centered management pearls that should be considered when managing these patients include identifying issues of housing security and adequate living space climate control (air conditioning and heating). A standard process to explore these during the discharge planning process will help avoid re-visits as well as better risk-stratify the appropriateness of discharging a patient. Identifying access to proper nutrition and food availability should also be discussed as there have been multiple studies that show a diet high in antioxidants and vitamins and low in sulfides decrease asthma exacerbations.[43]

Additionally, providing a patient-centered management approach is paramount. In urban settings, health literacy and access may be variable. An assessment of this will improve treatment and management decisions. Specifically, assessing previous therapies that have been successful as well as assessing the patient's understanding of the current illness are important ("What has worked in the past?" "Does this feel like previous episodes or when you were last admitted?"). Helping patients identify asthma triggers and initialing early and adequate treatment at home can empower patients in their own care and can diminish emergency room visits.

Patients who suffer from housing insecurity or live below the poverty line may not have the means to pay for medications and assuring access to treatment once they leave the emergency room is paramount. Ensuring that all patients can leave the ED with availability to bronchodilators and inhaled corticosteroids along with education related to proper medication administration can help increase medication adherence and diminish "bounce backs." Discussing alternatives with patients in case medications are too costly or pharmacies do not have medications stocked is an important part of the discharge process. Poor access to health care and overreliance on emergency facilities for asthma care (versus a primary care physician) has a negative impact on mortality, so primary care follow-up in a timely manner and return precautions must also be discussed prior to discharge.

Socioeconomic status such as household income, level of education, insurance status, and living below the poverty line are important determinants of health that have been shown to impact morbidity and mortality; as healthcare clinicians, it is important to acknowledge the impact of these factors to help breach their effects when it comes to access to treatment.

Vignette 1 Conclusion

The patient was evaluated in the ED and received nebulized albuterol and ipratropium bromide treatments as well as oral corticosteroids. His work of breathing, peak flow, and saturation improved, and there was no evidence of infections. The emergency physician explained to the grandmother that the likely culprit was multifactorial – weather, air quality factors related to the nearby building fire, as well as indoor factors related to the smoking neighbor, dogs in the building, as well as lack of adequate air conditioning. These factors are unique to the urban environment given close co-living quarters found in apartment complexes as well as local air quality issues that are problematic in socioeconomically depressed neighborhoods. Consulting with a social work team as well as housing authorities, Jonathan and his grandmother were able to find a more affordable housing situation in a smoke-free, pet-free building.

Vignette 2 Conclusion

The patient was evaluated in the ED and received nebulizer treatments as well as corticosteroids. His work of breathing, peak flow, and saturation improved, and there was no evidence of infections. The emergency physician explained to the patient that the likely culprit of the severe exacerbation was sudden exercise-induced vasospasm and the lack of an immediately available rescue device, along with the pollen from the recently blooming trees. If an inhaler was readily available, an ED visit might have been avoided. The abrasions noted were also cleaned and dressed, and in this case the patient was assessed for additional trauma that might be contributing to his respiratory distress. An appropriate physical exam was completed, electrocardiogram (EKG), lab studies, chest x-ray and a point of care ultrasound (POCUS) of the lungs were completed to assess for a clinically significant pneumothorax, cardiac concerns, and other issues. Access to rescue devices is a common theme for asthma patients in urban environments and discussing with patients appropriate strategies to ensure access at home, at work and school, and when on the go in parks, subways, and elsewhere is important.

Pro-Tips

- Asthma is an area of significant concern in EDs and has a host of problematic factors unique to the urban environment.
- Identifying that indoor, outdoor, and traffic-related pollution rates are higher in urban environments and acknowledging how they can negatively affect asthmatic patients is a crucial step to initiating early treatment and improving patient education.
- Exploring living situations as well as the financial situation of patients can positively impact opportunities for improved asthma care.
- Additional advocacy by emergency providers of the effects of urbanization on common disease entities, including asthma, is important.
- There are vast disparities in asthma management in urban populations.
- Early treatment and establishing proper medication accessibility is important to patient's adherence and overall control of exacerbations.

References

1. Marx JA, Rosen P. *Rosen's Emergency Medicine: Concepts and Clinical Practice.* 8th ed. Elsevier/Saunders, 2014.

2. Benjamin IJ, Griggs RC, Wing EJ, Fitz JG. *Andreoli and Carpenter's Cecil Essentials of Medicine.* 7th ed. Elsevier/Saunders, 2007.

3. Guarnieri M, Balmes JR. Outdoor air pollution and asthma. *Lancet*. 2014;383 (9928):1581–1592.

4. Center for Disease Control and Prevention. Most Recent National Asthma Data [Internet]. CDC; May 2022. Available from: www.cdc.gov/asthma/most_recent_national_asthma_data.htm

5. Pate C, Zahran H, Qin X, Johnson C, Hummelman E, Mailay J. Asthma surveillance – United States, 2006–2018. *MMWR Surveill Summ*. 2021;70(5):1–32.

6. World Health Organization. Asthma Fact Sheet. 2022. Available from: www.who.int /news-room/fact-sheets/detail/asthma

7. The International Study of Asthma and Allergies in Childhood Steering Committee.Worldwide variation in prevalence of symptoms of asthma, allergic rhinoconjunctivitis, and atopic eczema. *Lancet*. 1998;351(9111):1225–1232.

8. Institute for Health Metrics and Evaluation (IHME). Global Burden of Disease Compare Data Visualization. [Internet]. Institute for Health Metrics and Evaluations; 2020. Available from: https:// vizhub.healthdata.org/gbd-compare/

9. The Global Asthma Network. The Global Asthma Report. 2018. Auckland, New Zealand. Available from: http://globalasth mareport.org/

10. Asthma and Allergy Foundation of America. *Cost of Asthma on Society*. Arlington, VA. Available from: www .aafa.org/cost-of-asthma-on-society/#:~:te xt=Researchers%20think%20the%20yearly %20cost,States%20is%20around%20%245 6%20billion.&text=The%20direct%20costs %20make%20up,largest%20part%20of%20 that%20cost.&text=Indirect%20costs%20 make%20up%20%245.9%20billion (accessed March 3, 2023).

11. Nurmagambetov T, Kuwahara R, Garbe P. The economic burden of asthma in the United States, 2008–2013. *Ann Am Thorac Soc*. 2018;15(3):348–356. doi: 10.1513.

12. Diette GB, McCormack MC, Hansel NN, Breysse PN, Matsui EC. Environmental issues in managing asthma. *Respir Care*. 2008;53 (5):602–615; discussion 616–617.

13. Hoek G, Brunekreef B, Meijer R, Scholten A, Boleij J. Indoor nitrogen dioxide pollution and respiratory symptoms of schoolchildren. *Int Arch Occup Environ Health*. 1984;55(1):79–86.

14. Belanger K, Gent JF, Triche EW, Bracken MB, Leaderer BP. Association of indoor nitrogen dioxide exposure with respiratory symptoms in children with asthma. *Am J Respir Crit Care Med*. 2006;173(3):297–303.

15. Koenig JQ, Mar TF, Allen RW, Jansen K, Lumley T, Sullivan JH, Trenga CA, Larson TV, Liu LJS. Pulmonary effects of indoor- and outdoor-generated particles in children with asthma. *Environ Health Perpspect*. 2005;113(4):499–503.

16. Call RS, Smith TF, Morris E, Chapman MD, Platts-Mills TA. Risk factors for asthma in inner city children. *J Pediatr*. 1992;121(6):862–866.

17. Eggleston PA, Rosenstreich D, Lynn H, Gergen P, Baker D, Kattan M, Mortimer KM, Mitchell H, Ownby D, Slavin R, Malveaux F. Relationship of indoor allergen exposure to skin test sensitivity in inner-city children with asthma. *J Allergy Clin Immunol*. 1998;102(4 Pt 1):563–570.

18. Matsui EC, Wood RA, Rand C, Kanchanaraksa S, Swartz L, Curtin-Brosnan J, Eggleston PA. Cockroach allergen exposure and sensitization in suburban middle-class children with asthma. *JAllergy Clin Immunol*. 2003;112 (1):87–92.

19. Matsui EC, Simons E, Rand C, Butz A, Buckley TJ, Breysse P, Eggleston PA. Airborne mouse allergen in the homes of inner-city children with asthma. *JAllergy Clin Immunol*. 2005;115(2):358–363.

20. Perry T, Matsui E, Merriman B, Duong T, Eggleston PA. The prevalence of rat allergen in inner-city homes and its relationship to sensitization and asthma morbidity. *J Allergy Clin Immunol*. 2003;112(2):346–352.

21. United States Environmental Protection Agency. Ground Level Ozone Basics. 2022. www.epa.gov/ground-level-ozone-pollution/ground-level-ozone-basics#:~:text=air%20emission%20sources.-,How%20does%20ground-level%20ozone%20form%3F,volatile%20organic%20compounds%20(VOC)

22. Schultz ES, Litonjua AA, Melén E. Effects of long-term exposure to traffic-related air pollution on lung function in children. *Curr Allergy Asthma Rep J.* 2017;17:41.

23. Strosnider H, Kennedy C, Monti M, Yip F. Rural and urban differences in air quality, 2008–2012, and community drinking water quality, 2010–2015 – United States. *MMWR Surveill Summary* 2017;66(SS-13):1–10.

24. Malik HU, Kumar K, Frieri M. Minimal difference in the prevalence of asthma in the urban and rural environment. *Clin Med Insights Pediatrics.* 2012;6:33–39.

25. Holguin F. Traffic, outdoor air pollution, and asthma. *Immunol Allergy Clin North Am.* 2008;28:577–588.

26. United States Department of Transportation. Environment. 2020 May. Available from: www.transportation.gov/policy/transportation-policy/environment

27. D'Amato, G. Effects of climatic changes and urban air pollution on the rising trends of respiratory allergy and asthma. *MultidiscRespir Med.* 2011;6(1):28–37. https://doi.org/10.1186/2049-6958-6-1-28

28. Houston D, Basolo V, Yang D. Walkability, transit access, and traffic exposure for low-income residents with subsidized housing. *Am J Public Health.* 2013:103(4):673–678.

29. World Health Organization. Social Determinants of Health. 2022. Available from: www.who.int/health-topics/social-determinants-of-health#tab=tab_1

30. Cardet JC, Louisias M, King TS, Castro M, Codispoti CD, Dunn R, Engle L, Giles BL, Holguin F, Lima JJ, Long D, Lugogo N, Nyenhuis S, Ortega VE, Ramratnam S, Wechsler ME, Israel E, Phipatanakul W. Income as an independent risk factor for worse asthma outcome. *J Allergy Clin Immunol.* 2018;141(2):754–760.

31. Shrider E, Kollar M, Chen F, Semega J. Income and Poverty in the United States: 2020. United States Census Bureau. Income. 2021. Available from: www.census.gov/library/publications/2021/demo/p60-273.html

32. Smith Nightingale D, Wandner S. *Informal and Nonstandard Employment in the United States: Implications for Low Income Working Families.* The Urban Institute, 2011.

33. Grant T, Croce E, Matsui E. Asthma, and the social determinants of health. *Ann Allergy Asthma Immunol.* 2022;129(1):5–11.

34. Morrison AK, Glick A, Yin HS. Health literacy: implications for child health. *Pediatr Rev.* 2019;40(6):263–277.

35. Eagan T, Gulsvik A, Eide G, Bakke P. The effect of educational level on the incidence of asthma and respiratory symptoms. *Respir Med J.* 2004;98(8):730–736.

36. Emilio C, Mingotti C, Fiorin P, Lima L, Muniz RL, Bigotto LH, Marchi E, Ponte EV. Is a low level of education a limiting factor for asthma control in a population with access to pulmonologists and to treatment? *J Bras Pneumol.* 2019;45(1):e20180052.

37. Wright R, Mitchell H, Visness C, Cohen S, Stout J, Evans R, Gold D. Community violence and asthma morbidity: the Inner-City Asthma Study. *Am J Public Health.* 2004;94(4):625–632.

38. Landeo-Gutierrez J, Forno E, Miller G, Celedon J. Exposure to violence, psychosocial stress, and asthma. *Am J Respir Critical Care Med.* 2020;201(8):917–922.

39. Chiu YH, Coull BA, Sternthal MJ, Kloog I, Schwartz J, Cohen S, Wright RJ. Effects of prenatal community violence and ambient air pollution on childhood wheeze in an urban population. *J Allergy Clin Immunol.* 2014;133(3):713–722.

40. Cohen R, Canino G, Bird H, Celedón J. Violence, abuse, and asthma in Puerto Rican children. *Am J Respir Critical Care Med.* 2008;178:453–459.

41. Leigh S. *Racism Aggravated Treatment Resistant Asthma.* University of California San Francisco. 2017.

42. Darmon N, Drewnowski A. Contribution of food prices and diet cost to socioeconomic disparities in diet quality and health: a systematic review and analysis. *Nutr Rev.* 2015;73(10):643–660.

43. Litonjua AA. Dietary factors and the development of asthma. *Immunol Allergy Clin North Am.* 2008;28 (3):603–629. doi: 10.1016/j. iac.2008.03.005. PMID: 18572110; PMCID: PMC2536613.

44. Hing E, Hsiao C. US Department of Health and Human Services: State variability in supply of office based primary care providers. NCHS Data Brief, No. 151, May 2014.

45. Buchmueller TC, Jacobson M, Wold C. *How Far to the Hospital? The Effect of Hospital Closures on Access to Care.* NBER Working Paper No. 10700. National Bureau of Economic Research, 2004.

Physician/Patient Discordance

Tammy Jupic, Laura Smylie, and Elizabeth Dubey

Vignette 1

A 53-year-old female, primarily Bengali speaking, presents with pain. At triage, it is unclear where the pain is located due to a language barrier; gestures toward the abdomen and chest are equivocal. The resident working with you goes to evaluate the patient. He has trouble getting the interpreter phone to work so he uses a family member to obtain the history. The family member has limited English, too, but is slightly more fluent than the patient. The resident returns to divulge that the "gist" of the complaint is abdominal pain for a month, but the patient is not tender on exam. He is unable to obtain detailed information about review of systems. He then states, "I think it sounds like gastritis; we should order basic labs and maybe a lipase."

- Is the gathered history sufficient to proceed?

Vignette 2

An 82-year-old Chinese male is brought into the emergency department (ED) by his son. The son says that his father has been ill for five days. The patient had been complaining of abdominal pain and vomiting profusely. He has been trying to drink tea and boiling water to get better but "hasn't been able to keep anything down." The patient does not receive care from Western medicine-trained doctors and follows Eastern medicine only. Today, the son was finally able to convince the patient to present to the ED after he fainted. On exam, the patient has a large strangulated scrotal hernia that requires emergent surgery. However, he is refusing surgery, stating that he does not want any part of his body removed.

- How can this patient's cultural beliefs and values be reconciled with the clinician's recommendations?

Introduction

Discordance is the difference in traits between clinician and patient, whether it is secondary to language, religious differences, culture, race, or ethnicity. The term *concordance* indicates shared identities between physician and patient, which may make for more harmonious interpersonal interactions. Discordance between clinician and patient is a particular concern in urban EDs due to the cultural, racial, and linguistic plurality found in most large cities. Emergency clinicians are often the only or earliest points of contact with patients from marginalized groups; those removed from the healthcare system, those who face stigma, and those who hesitate to approach medical care. This discordance creates an environment for poor communication and misunderstanding between physician and patient. Discordance can manifest in many forms. This chapter will focus upon racial, linguistic, and cultural discordance, while discordances pertaining to sexual orientation and gender identity are addressed in the chapter on that topic.

Differing personal and healthcare experiences contribute to barriers, hindering effective clinical relationships. In the United States, there is distrust for the healthcare system by groups that have historically been marginalized and mistreated – often based on race. The 2018 National Healthcare Quality and Disparities Report found that patients identifying as Black/African American, American Indian, or Alaska Native received worse care in about 40% of the qualitative measures compared to White Caucasians.

Racial discordance is a particularly urban issue as rural America is less racially and ethnically diverse than urban areas. Although there are small statistical variances in percentages depending on the sources, generally Whites comprise nearly 80% of the rural population, compared with 58% percent of the urban population.[1] A 2018 report from USDA Economic Research Service shows that racial and ethnic minorities made up 22% of the rural population, compared to 43% of the urban population.[1]

Language discordance is also a common and well-known problem in medicine. When patients are unable to communicate with their physician, it can have deleterious or even devastating effects on both the care they receive and the rapport between the parties involved. This occurs commonly in EDs where there is often a lack of understanding or agreement about what was said due solely from a language mismatch. These language differences raise a practical barrier to obtaining a comprehensive history of present illness, past medical history, and even in obtaining an accurate physical exam.[2] The case of a man named Willie Ramirez is an example of morbidity that can arise from language discordance.[3] For Cuban Spanish speakers, *intoxicado* is a term that has multiple meanings, not necessarily associated with drug or alcohol *intoxication*. Providers assumed he had a drug overdose, thus, his diagnosis of intracerebral hemorrhage was delayed for two days. Language discordance can cause many problems that extend beyond communication alone, including longer wait times for medical services and increased stress on physicians. In 2017, 85% of immigrants to the United States resided in the top 100 metropolitan areas. In some US urban centers, non-English speakers comprise upwards of 38% of the patient population. This is not unique to the United States: in the 2016 Australian census, 22% of households did not speak English as the primary language, and 41% of households in Sydney's urban center did not speak English as the primary language.[4] According to 2016 Canadian census data, nearly 7.6 million Canadians speak a language other than the two Canadian mother tongues (English and French) at home, an increase from 2011 of 14.5% (nearly one million people). Per census data, this correlates to 22.3% of the Canadian population. Not surprisingly, most immigrant language speakers were in Canadian urban centers.[5] Although language alone is not the only factor that contributes to discordance, it is often an initially high barrier to surmount.

The conflict between different cultures is often more nuanced than race or language. The practices of one culture can differ greatly from another, even when they are living in the same area and speaking mutually understandable languages; this occurs for many reasons including religious beliefs that may not agree with those built into Western Culture. Many times, these differences go unnoticed by physicians, especially when language is also a factor in communication. Physicians sometimes show less empathy when they are from discordant cultures and patients tend to be less satisfied with their care when part of a discordant dyad.[6,7] There are likely differing expectations and values that contribute to this perceived (and likely actual) worse care. In many cultures, people do not contradict an authority figure, such as an ED physician, and this too complicates care. When women from some Middle Eastern cultures seek care in the ED, they often strongly prefer women physicians, and may even decline examination by male physicians as a consequence of their culture. Our women clinicians often feel burdened by this preference, and our male clinicians can get frustrated by their inability to properly examine their patients.

Although the incidence of explicit and systemic discrimination in US healthcare is declining, there remains implicit bias. "Bias" has many meanings, but broadly, it is the negative assessment of a group and its members in comparison to another group. As healthcare clinicians, we must recognize our own biases and strive to combat those prejudices and partialities in order to effectively and compassionately join patients from all walks of life in their journey to health. This unconscious discrimination is a product of many things, discordance being one. Urban emergency physicians are often the only or earliest points of contact with patients from marginalized groups, those removed from the healthcare system, those who face stigma, and those who hesitate to approach medical care. Arguably, the discordance between us as clinicians and our patients in urban EDs is greater than any other area of the healthcare system. As we work to make the healthcare system a more equitable place for all who seek care, our EDs are the imperfect laboratories where we acutely experience the difficulties of putting our ideals into practice.

Excellent practice of emergency medicine in the urban setting requires much more than medical knowledge and clinical acumen; it is necessary to develop interpersonal skills that allow for the creation of rapport and trust with patients from various cultural, ethnic, and racial backgrounds. Patients and physicians can have very different backgrounds and experiences both in and out of the healthcare realm, and through intentional efforts, can create good outcomes for patients regardless of discordance.

Physician/Patient Discordance in the Emergency Department

Discordance between urban ED physicians and their patients is common.

The Association of American Medical College (AAMC) data from the 2019–2020 emergency medicine resident applicant pool revealed that clinicians identifying as White were still the majority at 67.6%. Of a total of 5921 active emergency resident physicians polled, 0.9% were American Indian, 18.2% were Asian or Pacific Islander, and 5.9% were Black. Approximately 8.8% were Hispanic.[8] In the broader AAMC physician workforce data (albeit, 14% of poll participants did not elucidate their race), the vast majority of current practicing physicians identified as White (over 50%); approximately 17% identified as Asian, nearly 6% identified as Hispanic, and 5% identified as Black or African American. Reassuringly, review of the available AAMC data from 2010 (nearly one decade prior to the aforementioned data) revealed that the physician workforce diversity has improved: between 1978 and 2008, three quarters of all practicing medical school graduates were White. Meanwhile, a combined 12.3% of the American physician workplace was a combination of American Indians, Blacks, Hispanics, and Latinos. Then, Asians comprised 12.8% of minority physicians and Blacks comprised 6.3%.[9]

The American physician workforce is more diverse than ever before; however, it has not risen in stride with the rise of minorities in our population.[10] As a consequence of the physician demographic landscape, discordance between patient and physician is inevitable in urban centers despite efforts toward diversity. Urban EDs have the unavoidable responsibility of becoming a confluence for diverse interactions. Recognize that in many urban cities, non-English speakers exceed a quarter of the region's population. Underrepresented American minorities comprise 30% of the American population, yet based on 2018 AAMC data, only approximately 20% of all emergency clinicians are minorities.[11,12] This is fraught with challenges, especially when patient demographics are dissimilar to clinicians, leading to discordance in physician–patient encounters. This phenomenon of discordance is problematic because physician behavior implicitly alters based on a patient's identity, dependent on whatever degree of difference both exhibit.

Race

Racial discordance in medicine can be objectively obvious, yet can have elusive repercussions in everyday medical interactions. When a physician and patient come from different racial backgrounds, there is also the risk of cultural, societal, or socioeconomic incongruity. This is in addition to possible inherent bias on the part of the physician and underlying distrust from the patient due to racial differences.

Data suggest that when physician and patient encounters have concordance, outcomes generally improve. In America's 50 largest cities, census data demonstrate consistently more diversified populations: in the year 2000, 42% of the population was White; in 2010, 39%, and in 2020, 36%.[13] In the city of Detroit, over three quarters of the population identifies as Black: notably, based on available data regarding physicians in Detroit, the percentage of ED physicians who identify as Black in Detroit is approximately 6%. Even if patients desire a more concordant clinician–patient relationship, it is not possible in urban centers.

In a recent study of California physicians, it was found that African American and Hispanic physicians were more likely than White physicians to care for minority patients and those who were uninsured or covered by Medicaid.[14] Another survey asked participants for several interpersonal care aspects and Black patients had significantly lower mean scores for trust of healthcare clinicians compared to White.[15] In fact, this was a predictor for lower levels of trust. Historically, White physicians demonstrated less empathy and non-verbal attention toward Black patients or a more "biomedical" communication style. Records also highlight that White physicians previously spent less time educating or answering questions.[16] In the United Kingdom, recent survey data demonstrate that Bangladeshi patients experience the most dissatisfaction with their health care compared with other races.

Indeed, another systematic review that assessed racially discordant interactions of clinicians and implicit bias elucidated a relationship between level of implicit bias and lower quality of care: it was noted that physicians with higher levels of implicit bias used first-person plural pronouns and anxiety-related words more often than physicians with lower levels of bias who had engaged in discordant interactions.[17] Furthermore, in other studies, minority patients receive lower interpersonal care than White patients, no matter the physician's identity. Recall that frequently, ED physicians are the only or earliest physician interactions for minority patients or patients who delay medical care and consequently, these interactions perpetuate a cycle of discouragement with healthcare.

Although there are many approaches to race, sociology describes two popular approaches: color-blindness and multiculturalism. Color-blindness focuses on excluding race in judgment as a means to limit discrimination. As popular as this perspective is, physicians – although not explicitly acknowledging race – can still bear unconscious biases toward minorities and appear less engaged. According to some studies, balancing the exterior presentation of trying to appear unprejudiced can cause Whites to "appear more uncomfortable, more anxious, and less friendly during interracial interactions." On the other hand, multiculturalism emphasizes the importance of acknowledging and empowering all races, celebrating diversity, and acknowledging demographic shifts.[18] Studies show that minorities prefer this approach, as this allows physicians to acknowledge minority patients and learn of their perspectives. More empathetic active listening is required with multicultural approaches. However, research has demonstrated that this approach might cause minorities to be valued based on their minority status and does little to promote positive group relations.

Language/Linguistics

Recall that language concordance occurs when there is fluency between the physician and the patient's preferred language; it is a known truth that communication is key to optimal patient care outcomes, even an improvement to outcomes. After all, proper emergency medicine care is predicated on a thorough history and physical. This is also seen with regards to preventative services after physician–patient interactions: a recent systematic review determined that generally, limited English proficiency (LEP) in an English-dominated system demonstrated diminished access to preventive services, cancer screening, and worse healthcare quality and outcomes.[19] Concordance relationship outcomes include fewer unasked questions, better medication compliance, and fewer ED visits. Other studies show that patients are more satisfied by concordant physician–patient encounters.[14] In fact, another study noted that discordant relationships resulted in lower likelihood of disclosing mental health needs.[20] There is also the question of proper informed consent with the use of language interpreter services – or lack thereof. Sometimes, busy emergency medicine physicians perform a more cursory examination and history in the expectation that they (or someone else) will later grab an interpreter and perform a more detailed history and physical later – but the moment might never arrive, all too painfully obvious in resource-scarce urban EDs in a post-COVID era.

In patient interactions, clinicians sometimes do not utilize a patient translator, due to external limitations of resources or time or energy. Perhaps a patient presentation is so emergent that there is no time to obtain a translator. Physicians are time- and resource-limited, often driven by Relative Value Units (RVU) and external metrics (initially designed with good intent but oftentimes cumbersome in execution for clinicians). Effective and functional communication is inherently more demanding when barriers prevail– logistical or language. Software or Internet-related barriers to video/telephone interpretation, long wait times due to inadequate staffing or availability, and even interpretive inaccuracies can cause further communication lapses. There is time and labor associated with obtaining interpreter services, frustrating in a bustling urban ED. Unfortunately, obtaining proper translation, the back-and-forth and childhood telephone game nature of interpreter dialogue, and the time required for history clarification indubitably increase the patient-care interaction. Less than ideal interactions among patients with limited English proficiency were more common with language-discordant physicians. A national survey revealed that 33% of American residents utilized a child under 12 years of age for interpretation.[21]

Using lay persons for translation, including hospital staff lacking specific training, can result in inadequate communication. Clinicians and patients can be misled into a false sense of understanding, which has been demonstrated to contribute to worse results or errors.[22] Studies have even demonstrated that bilingual physicians still have substantial risk for lapses in understanding or communication. This is in part possible because a physician's multilinguality is not always equivalent to the patient's language fluency. Nearly half of all encounters in another study resulted in serious miscommunication impacting the patient's care by either undermining the patient's symptoms or ineffectively communicating the patient's concerns.[23] The case of Willie Ramirez is a frequently mentioned example of adverse patient outcome in the setting of mistranslation with use of a lay person. Furthermore, diction is less readily available or nuanced when basic words like "pain" are difficult to elicit, let alone whether the pain is "burning," "shooting," or "stabbing." However, interpreters have their own limitations, because in most countries, professional interpreter services strive to be a neutral language translator, not necessarily interpretive of inflection, emotion, or intention. Certain details and gestures are lost over phone translation. Patients in a bustling, loud ED, cannot hear the translator phone properly, which is exacerbated if the patient is elderly. Furthermore, interpreter services are inconsistent. Because of this, cost to the patient and medical healthcare system can be increased, as the emergency physician must catch a broader differential net to ensure patient safety: in a study that assessed non-English speakers and abdominal pain, non-English speakers had more tests ordered.[24] In a separate study that assessed pediatric ED encounters, there was an increased charge for diagnostic testing and greater number of admissions.[25]

Ultimately, several studies have shown that despite current availability of interpreter services, there is low utilization of these services. Interacting with LEP patients requires modeling good behavior. Students who are impressionable recollect patient care interactions based on resident and attending interactions. With regard to perceived values, good bedside manners with the use of interpreter services appeared to be less valuable than clinical knowledge alone, and there is no reward for students to utilize interpreter services.

To reduce the cognitive burden in such an atmosphere, stereotyping in the ED is a common tool to mitigate limited resources.[16] When languages or races are concordant, clinical visits tend to be more patient-centric, are longer, and characterized by a more positive impression of the encounter.[26] American studies have shown that physicians were less in-depth toward symptoms of non–English-speaking patients.[27] This is only evident with the effective use of good translation services. Only by concordant understanding of the patient's ideas and verbalized comprehension of their disease can the physician truly understand the patient's beliefs and "social attachments" to the disease, presumptions of the treatment plan, or end target of disease management.

Culture

Culture is the belief and identity system a person to which a person subscribes. It can impact values regarding disease and treatment. Various studies argue for cultural sensitivity or treating patients equally regardless of culture. However, this is not sensitive care and specific needs of each patient should be addressed in the urban ED. One study noted physicians avoided discussing race or ethnicity, and this "strategic color-blindness" has been shown to worsen interactions: other studies have shown that explicitly recognizing culture reduces bias and improves clinician perspectives.

Cultural discordance is correlated with more passive patient–physician encounters among migrant and ethnic minority patients: compared to native-born patients, they "ask fewer questions, take fewer initiatives, and are less involved in the decision-making process."[28]

Notably, not all patients have Western biomedical ideologies. In current medicine, Western practices are believed to be the most modern and ergo the best for patient care. In some cultures, this Western superiority complex is hubristic and demeaning to those who believe in alternative medicine (such as with Indigenous Peoples) or Eastern practices. Some cultures vary vastly regarding physician perceptions. Rather than a collective partnership, as much of Western medicine is trending toward, some cultures still maintain a hierarchical impression of medicine: the physician knows best or knows all and does not require further information from the patient. This was a contributing factor to the fatal assumption in Willie Ramirez's case. He was a dedicated athlete who did not partake in drugs, but when the physician assumed the Spanish term *intoxicado* meant "intoxicated," the family did not contradict this. There are also differences in communication styles and values especially when pertaining to medical decision making. Sometimes, emergency medicine physicians label the patient as a "poor historian" and move on without time to delve into the patient's presentation. In documentation, this can make the patient appear culpable for their perceived poor insight or health status.

For example, Islamic cultural norms result in frequently quiescent patients who oftentimes strive to not impede clinical care. Frequently, Muslim patients do not verbalize their problems and expect physicians to anticipate their needs. There is a strong love of God and family and a respect for physicians.[29] For Islamic patients, touching the opposite gender is oftentimes discouraged, which can be difficult logistically in an ED.

Negative Outcomes of Discordance

Discordance has negative impacts on patient care. In a 1990 study, it was noted that Hispanics with isolated long bone fractures were twice as likely than non-Hispanic Whites to receive no pain medication at a single-site ED in California.[30] In that study, it was also noted that non-Hispanic White patients were more likely to speak English and be insured and suffer non-occupational injuries.[30] Another multicenter study found that Black/African American and Hispanic ED patients under an involuntary psychiatric evaluation hold experience higher rates of physical restraint use compared to their White/Caucasian counterparts.[31] This disparity is also paralleled in the United Kingdom, where Black patients are more likely to be detained under the Mental Health Act than are White patients.[20] In the United Kingdom and in the United States, Black women are still more likely to die peripartum than White women; in the most recent summary provided by the United Kingdom, Black minority women are four times more likely to die than White women and Asian minorities are twice as likely to die.[32] Emergency department analgesia for children with acute appendicitis in Israeli government hospitals is markedly low. In one study assessing patient–nurse ethnic discordance at Israeli government hospitals, it was found that Jewish and Arab nurses gave proportionally less analgesia to the opposite group.[33]

Limited language proficiency impairs patient understanding, limits accessible care, and poorly impacts medical compliance. These barriers are also affiliated with increased hospital duration and decreased health history. Discordance, in general, has led to adverse events and mortality in patient care. In one Australian study, LEP was an independent predictor of prolonged symptom-to-door time with regard to primary percutaneous coronary intervention for ST-elevation myocardial infarction.[34] The authors speculate whether hesitation is due to cost concerns or cultural reasons. Perhaps it is an inability to effectively communicate urgency or details. Patients with LEP are reluctant to hail emergent services like ambulance transfer for reasons such as cost concerns, language barriers, and even cultural reasons. Notably, minority patients tend to present to the ED later in disease processes, thus resulting in more emergent or morbid outcomes, as they did not receive adequate primary care. Morbidity includes diabetic ketoacidosis or even amputation. Other studies note that LEP patients are nearly a quarter more likely to return to the ED within 72 hours. Language barriers are also associated with increased adverse events and safety risks.[23] Studies have shown that LEP patients had less satisfaction, differing rates of diagnostics, less explanation from clinicians, and less follow-up than their more English-proficient counterparts.[35] Even after statistical adjustment for insurance status and income, racial and ethnic minorities presenting to the ED were noted to receive lower-quality care. Although there is less explicit physician bias, physicians still have implicit bias that affects patients beyond the physician–patient encounter, ultimately reducing trust and medication compliance.

A study analyzing adverse event data from six hospitals over seven months noted that approximately 49% of LEP patient adverse events had some physical harm compared to 29% of English-proficient adverse events.[23] These adverse events toward patients with LEP were more likely to be from communication errors. However, from 2003, another study noted that interpreter services were underutilized.

Reasons for Hope

Results of discordant language, racial, and cultural physician–patient interactions are not all negative. Despite the plethora of evidence suggesting adverse events and challenges associated with discordance, several studies do demonstrate that ultimately, clinical emergency medicine has many algorithmic attributes. Although clinical gestalt plays a large role in clinical decision making, much of emergency training is based on protocols, criteria, metrics, and guidelines, mitigating cognitive and implicit bias. Evidence-based guidelines have paved the way for equitable care without turning a blind eye to discordance. Many national standards and legislations have limited discrepancies in clinical practice. The American Accreditation Council for Graduate Medical Education (ACGME) has a set list of criteria each emergency medicine program must fulfill. These set aspects of training can save lives, ameliorate disease, and properly disposition patients, regardless of physician–patient discordance or concordance. The ACGME explicitly emphasizes that residents "must demonstrate competence in [. . .] respect and responsiveness to diverse patient populations, including but not limited to diversity in gender, age, culture, race, religion, disabilities, national origin, socioeconomic status, and sexual orientation."[36] In a recent review, it was determined that regardless of specialty, physicians did demonstrate an implicit bias for White patients; however, this bias did not appear to affect clinical decision making.[37]

Although the results of the aforementioned Australian study suggest that prolonged symptom-to-door time exists for LEP patients, percutaneous coronary intervention for these LEP myocardial infarction patients does not lead to worse 30-day mortality, which is ultimately the goal. In the aforementioned study that assessed laboratory studies and imaging ordered for abdominal pain, it also demonstrated that there was no statistically significant difference with regard to chest pain studies.[24] An Australian study assessed chest pain between culturally and linguistically diverse patients and non-culturally and linguistically diverse patients and similar to a previously mentioned study in the United States, there were no significant differences in the number of laboratory or clinical investigations carried out between groups or significant differences in analgesia, ED length of stay or hospital admission rate.[38] Several studies have demonstrated that once the patient is in the health care trajectory beyond the ED doors, LEP does not affect in-hospital mortality.[39]

To mitigate the negative effects of discordance, several tangible advances have been enacted. In December 2018, the Amsterdam Center for Health Communication organized a symposium that discussed the current state of medicine and innovations to improve intercultural communication in healthcare.[28] Questions posed include how language barriers in intercultural health communication could be mitigated. Although sometimes underutilized, translation resources are federally mandated: The Affordable Care Act Section 1557 mandates all healthcare institutions receiving federal funds provide qualified medical interpreters to patients of limited English proficiency.

Emphasis is placed on cultural and linguistic competence now in recognition of former and perpetuating disparities. Studies suggest that professional developmental series in cultural and linguistic competence has improved attitudes and skills. Personal responsibility for the need for cultural competency in the urban setting is pivotal to improving patient care. Although programs are slowly adopting curricula that address implicit biases, many are eager to adopt one. There are gaps in "content," "quality," and "expertise of the presenters." In the United States, state-by-state licensing boards and medical schools have begun adopting implicit bias training into licensure and curricula. In the wake of recent social events, the American Medical Association pledged to address medical racism and adopted policy that acknowledged racism and unconscious bias perpetuation of disparities and health care delivery. The Agency for Healthcare Research and Quality, a division of the US Department of Health and Human Services, has developed training to improve patient safety, including the development of a LEP program.[40]

A recent survey was sent to the director of every accredited Emergency Medicine residency program in the US.[41] Of the 168 programs, approximately 43% responded. 68% included cultural competence education and of these, 90% were structured didactics. For those 50 programs, 43 included race and ethnicity didactics and only 20 discussed LEP. Reassuringly, 93% of the respondents were interested in a universal open-source cultural competency curriculum.

Another important means to address language discordance is to reconceptualize the role of interpreter: rather than translating speech verbatim, interpreters ought to be collaborators and partners with the patient, especially with regard to cultural nuance. One popular translation service highlights the importance of language proficiency and successful completion of training courses and years of experience; however, there is no emphasis on being culturally sensitive or sensitive to patient emotion or wishes. More studies are necessary to evaluate the impact of multimedia tools to educate patients or facilitate communication and public health advocacy; however, there is great potential to enact improvements in patient care in this digital age.

Ultimately, it is imperative that emergency medicine continues to diversify the physician pool. The first female physician in America graduated in 1849. The first non-White physician graduated in 1837. Several leaps and strides have been made, but as highlighted earlier, the journey to more representative medicine is still ongoing. In 2009, the Liaison Committee on Medical Education introduced two standards aimed at achieving institutional diversity and investing in pipeline programs to increase the number of qualified diverse applicants. However, research indicates that these efforts have made only a marginal difference in advancing diversity in medical education.

Partnership between physician and patient regardless of concordance or discordance is an important mentality to establish as emergency medicine physicians. Emergency medical care should emphasize patient preferences and thus improve patient outcomes and increase patient satisfaction. Partnership, or shared decision-making practice, is known to positively impact patient satisfaction and compliance.[22] In addition, the emphasis on recent medical education and practices to incorporate humanistic medicine has fueled more equitable care despite discordance: by remembering a patient is human, it is easier to care on a more personal level. Combating discordance is an evolving sphere, but with more concerted awareness and efforts, there is promise for improved patient outcomes regardless of identities.

Cultural competence is not a one-time event, but rather an ongoing journey. Constant self-reflection and humility to accept when one is wrong are key in developing this skill. Additionally, it is important to understand that there is always more to learn – no one can ever be an expert on all cultures. As the world becomes increasingly connected, it is crucial that emergency medicine clinicians strive to continuously improve upon this skill. Addressing discordance in emergency medicine is critical to providing quality care for all patients. By recognizing one's own biases and educating oneself on patient cultures, races, and languages, better care and relationships can be formed.

Vignette 1 Conclusion

There are several drawbacks to continuing with the restricted history. It's probable that significant details have been overlooked. Two genuine issues could arise as a result of this: one is that the workup will not be thorough, and the other is that the physician may miss a vital diagnosis because he or she will take a "shotgun" approach rather than doing a targeted evaluation. It is important to gather an accurate history in any patient who has the capacity to provide it. First, try to troubleshoot the interpreter phone problem. If it's not working, there are on-line interpreter apps that may be used, although the quality can vary. You can also look to your ED staff for help. Does anyone speak her language? If not, does she have any other family members available by phone who could help ask more pointed questions?

After a couple of calls, the patient is able to get her youngest daughter on the phone who speaks English fluently. After obtaining more of a history, you gather that her pain also involves her chest, so you add on a cardiac workup. Her ECG shows non-specific abnormalities, but the troponin is positive, and she receives cardiac catheterization that shows nearly 100% right coronary artery (RCA) stenosis. She is stented and able to be discharged the next day.

Vignette 2 Conclusion

Although many modern East Asians do not consciously follow Confucian beliefs, certain modern beliefs are still influenced by cultural values including filial piety and the necessity of "dying intact" as a form of respecting ancestors. This makes many East Asians less inclined to be organ donors or blood donors. In the ED, it is important to be aware of these values and to be respectful when discussing organ donation, blood transfusion, or surgery resulting in tissue removal with patients and families. Clinicians must also be culturally humble and remember that their own cultural values may not be held by all patients. In this case, the clinician could offer to speak to the patient and his son about the significance of this surgical procedure and how it may be viewed as an act of filial piety. Only then will the patient and physician be able to make an informed decision about his care together.

Pro-Tips

Discordance in the ED creates an environment for poor communication and misunderstanding to grow between physician and patient. It can also result in inferior care and worse health outcomes for patients. However, there are numerous ways physicians can take actions to address discordance in their ED.

- Take an active approach to recognize your own cultural framework. Project Implicit offers multiple Implicit Bias Tests, allowing users to evaluate their associations with various items ranging from race to social class.

- Partake in formal bias training on how to effectively communicate with patients from diverse backgrounds in order to facilitate better patient care. There are available resources online including the US Department of Health and Human Services-developed program TeamSTEPPS that has a dedicated course for LEP.[40]

- As an emergency medicine physician, modeling the use of effective and thorough interpretive services is essential for future generations of physicians. While arranging the interpreter can be cumbersome, it will go a long way toward ensuring that patients get the right treatment.

- Physicians may not be the best representatives of their respective urban populations, but other staff members are and can be essential. While formal interpretative services are essential and irreplaceable, the use of staff for communication has a role.

- Consider ways in which mobile applications and other online resources can also provide patients with information about their condition, as well as instructions on how to care for themselves at home.

References

1. Cromartie J. Rural America at a glance 2018 edition. *Economic Information Bulletin* No. EIB-200. 2018.

3. Bridges AJ, Andrews AR, 3rd, Deen TL. Mental health needs and service utilization by Hispanic immigrants residing in mid-southern United States. *J Transcult Nurs.* 2012;23(4):359–368.

3. www.healthaffairs.org/do/10.1377/fore front.20081119.000463/

4. Statistics ABo. 2016 Census QuickStats. 2016.

5. Canada S. An increasingly diverse linguistic profile: Corrected data from the 2016 Census. *The Daily*; 2017.

6. Schouten BC, Meeuwesen L. Cultural differences in medical communication: a review of the literature. *Patient Educ Counsel.* 2006;64(1–3):21–34.

7. Takeshita J, Wang S, Loren AW, Mitra N, Shults J, Shin DB, Sawinsky DL.

Association of racial/ethnic and gender concordance between patients and physicians with patient experience ratings. *JAMA Netw Open.* 2020;3(11): e2024583.

8. Association of American Medical Colleges. *Report on Residents.* AAMC, 2020.

9. Association of American Medical Colleges. *Diversity in the Physician Workforce: Facts & Figures 2010.* AAMC, 2010.

10. Lett E, Orji WU, Sebro R. Declining racial and ethnic representation in clinical academic medicine: a longitudinal study of 16 US medical specialties. *PLoS One.* 2018;13(11):e0207274.

11. Association of American Medical Colleges. *Diversity in Medicine: Facts and Figures 2019.* AAMC, 2019.

12. Association of American Medical Colleges. *Diversity in Medicine: Facts and Figures 2019.* AAMC, 2019.

13. Parker K HJ, Brown A, Fry R, Cohn DV, Igielnik R. *What Unites and Divides Urban, Suburban, and Rural Communities*. Pew Research Center, 2018.

14. Blanchard JC, Haywood YC, Scott C. Racial and ethnic disparities in health: an emergency medicine perspective. *Acad Emerg Med*. 2003;10(11):1289–1293.

15. Lee JS, Tamayo-Sarver J, Kinneer P, Hobgood C. Association between patient race/ethnicity and perceived interpersonal aspects of care in the emergency department. *J Natl Med Assoc*. 2008;100(1):79–85.

16. Cooper LA, Beach MC, Johnson RL, Inui TS. Delving below the surface. Understanding how race and ethnicity influence relationships in health care. *J Gen Intern Med*. 2006;21(Suppl 1):S21–27.

17. Hagiwara N, Slatcher RB, Eggly S, Penner LA. Physician racial bias and word use during racially discordant medical interactions. *Health Commun*. 2017;32 (4):401–408.

18. West TV, Schoenthaler A. Color-blind and multicultural strategies in medical settings. *Social Iss Policy Rev*. 2018;11(1):124–158.

19. DuBard CA, Gizlice Z. Language spoken and differences in health status, access to care, and receipt of preventive services among US Hispanics. *Am J Public Health*. 2008;98(11):2021–2028.

20. August KJ, Nguyen H, Ngo-Metzger Q, Sorkin DH. Language concordance and patient–physician communication regarding mental health needs. *J Am Geriatr Soc*. 2011;59(12):2356–2362.

21. Kenison TC, Madu A, Krupat E, Ticona L, Vargas IM, Green AR. Through the veil of language: exploring the hidden curriculum for the care of patients with limited English proficiency. *Acad Med*. 2017;92(1):92–100.

22. Soled D. Language and cultural discordance: barriers to improved patient care and understanding. *J Patient Exp*. 2020;7(6):830–832.

23. Divi C, Koss RG, Schmaltz SP, Loeb JM. Language proficiency and adverse events in US hospitals: a pilot study. *Int J Qual Health Care*. 2007;19(2):60–67.

24. Waxman MA, Levitt MA. Are diagnostic testing and admission rates higher in non-English-speaking versus English-speaking patients in the emergency department? *Ann Emerg Med*. 2000;36(5):456–461.

25. Rogers AJ, Delgado CA, Simon HK. The effect of limited English proficiency on admission rates from a pediatric ED: stratification by triage acuity. *Am J Emerg Med*. 2004;22(7):534–536.

26. Cooper LA, Roter DL, Johnson RL, Ford DE, Steinwachs DM, Powe NR. Patient-centered communication, ratings of care, and concordance of patient and physician race. *Ann Intern Med*. 2003;139 (11):907–915.

27. Cooper LA. Health disparities. Toward a better understanding of primary care patient-physician relationships. *J Gen Intern Med*. 2004;19(9):985–986.

28. Schouten BC, Cox A, Duran G, Kerremans K, Banning LK, Lahdidioui A, van den Muijsenbergh M, Schinkel S, Sungur H, Suurmond J, Zendedel R, Krystallidou D. Mitigating language and cultural barriers in healthcare communication: toward a holistic approach. *Patient Educ Counsel*. 2020; S0738-3991(20)30242-1.

29. Ezenkwele UA, Roodsari GS. Cultural competencies in emergency medicine: caring for Muslim-American patients from the Middle East. *J Emerg Med*. 2013;45 (2):168–174.

30. Todd KH, Samaroo N, Hoffman JR. Ethnicity as a risk factor for inadequate emergency department analgesia. *JAMA*. 1993;269(12):1537–1539.

31. Carreras Tartak JA, Brisbon N, Wilkie S, Sequist TD, Aisiku IP, Raja A, Macias-Konstantopoulos WL. Racial and ethnic disparities in emergency department restraint use: a multicenter retrospective analysis. *Acad Emerg Med*. 2021;28 (9):957–965.

32. MBRRACE-UK. *Saving Lives, Improving Mothers' Care: Lessons Learned to Inform Maternity Care from the UK and Ireland Confidential Enquiries into Maternal*

Deaths and Morbidity 2015–17. Oxford Population Health, 2019.

33. Shavit I, Jacob R, Friedman N, Capua T, Klein A, Chistyakov I, Moldaver I, Krupik D, Munchak I, Abozaid S, Rimon A, Meirson G, Leiba R, Cohen DM. Effect of patient and nurse ethnicity on emergency department analgesia for children with appendicitis in Israeli government hospitals. *Eur J Pain*. 2018;22(10):1711–1717.

34. Biswas S, Seman M, Cox N, Neil C, Brennan A, Dinh D, Walton A, Chan W, Lefkovits J, Reid C, Stub D. Impact of limited English proficiency on presentation and outcomes of patients undergoing primary percutaneous coronary intervention for ST-elevation myocardial infarction. *Intern Med J*. 2018;48 (4):457–461.

35. Ramirez D, Engel KG, Tang TS. Language interpreter utilization in the emergency department setting: a clinical review. *J Health Care Poor Underserved*. 2008;19(2):352–362.

36. Accreditation Council for Graduate Medical Education. *ACGME Program Requirements for Graduate Medical Education in Emergency Medicine*. ACGME, 2021.

37. Dehon E, Weiss N, Jones J, Faulconer W, Hinton E, Sterling S. A systematic review of the impact of physician implicit racial bias on clinical decision making. *Acad Emerg Med*. 2017;24(8):895–904.

38. Ngai KM, Grudzen CR, Lee R, Tong VY, Richardson LD, Fernandez A. The association between limited English proficiency and unplanned emergency department revisit within 72 hours. *Ann Emerg Med*. 2016;68(2):213–221.

39. John-Baptiste A, Naglie G, Tomlinson G, Alibhai SM, Etchells E, Cheung A, Kapral M, Gold WL, Abrams H, Bacchus M, Krahn M. The effect of English language proficiency on length of stay and in-hospital mortality. *J Gen Intern Med*. 2004;19(3):221–228.

40. Agency for Healthcare Research and Quality. *Improving Patient Safety Systems for Patients With Limited English Proficiency: A Guide for Hospitals*. The Disparities Solutions Center, Mongan Institute for Health Policy, Massachusetts General Hospital, 2012.

41. Mechanic OJ, Dubosh NM, Rosen CL, Landry AM. Cultural competency training in emergency medicine. *J Emerg Med*. 2017;53(3):391–396.

Further Reading

1. US Department of Health and Human Services. *2018 National Healthcare Quality and Disparities Report*. AHRQ, 2019.

2. Vogel L. Broken trust drives native health disparities. *CMAJ*. 2015;187(1): E9–E10.

Chapter 10

LGBTQIA+ Care

Nicholas Avitabile

Vignette

A 24-year-old transgender female registers with the triage nurse in the waiting room of the emergency department (ED). You overhear some of the security guards making fun of her, stating she is not a "real" woman, and that she is a "freak." You recognize her as a transgender patient who was assigned male at birth but now identifies as female and is status-post gender affirmation surgery. You hear her crying, and she starts to get up to leave.

- What is the best way to reassure her that she will receive good care in the ED?
- What kind of disciplinary action, if any, should be taken against the security guards?
- What are some measures you can take to avoid similar events from happening in the first place?

Introduction

LGBTQIA+ patients have historically faced discrimination, effects of implicit bias, and failures of cultural competence while in the ED. It has been suggested that these shortcomings are rooted in microaggressions, or "brief, nuanced, and often unintentional slights and offenses that underlie verbal and nonverbal communication."[1] Specifically, "heteronormative" microaggressions make LGBTQIA+ patients feel that their identities, experiences, and relationships are abnormal, pathological, unexpected, unwelcome, or shameful. These negative messages undermine patient–provider trust and may lead LGBTQIA+ individuals to avoid seeking care.[2]

Dedicated training in cultural competency is a common component of onboarding in hospitals and EDs, although many clinicians remain uncomfortable caring for LGBTQIA+ patients. One study of emergency medicine (EM) residents found that 25% were not comfortable taking histories and physicals from lesbian, gay, and bisexual patients, and 42% were not comfortable with transgender patients.[3] It is clear that formally educating clinicians in cultural competency increases their cultural competence level, which in turn increases patient satisfaction.[4]

In addition to training clinicians, EDs should demonstrate that they support and welcome LGBTQIA+ patients. Many EDs and clinics place LGBTQIA+ flags and welcome signs in the waiting area; such signage is unassociated with any political agenda and should not be taken as antithetical to any political or religious beliefs. Also, preferred names and pronouns should be solicited and utilized, and gender-neutral bathrooms should be available. Gender-related terminology is given in Table 10.1.

Table 10.1 Gender-Related Terminology

LGBTQIA+	Stands for lesbian, gay, bisexual, transgender, queer, intersex, asexual, or ally +. The "+" signifies that anything else not specifically listed as part of the acronym may also be represented
Affirmed gender	When one's gender identity is validated by others as authentic
Agender	Person who identifies as genderless or outside the gender continuum
Cisgender	A person whose gender identity and/or expression aligns with their sex assigned at birth (antonym: Transgender)
Cross-dressing	Wearing of clothes typically associated with another gender; the term transvestite can be considered pejorative and should not be used
Cultural humility	Concept of not projecting one's own personal experiences and preconceptions of identity onto the experiences and identities of others
Differences of sex development	Congenital conditions characterized by nuanced chromosomal, gonadal, or anatomic sex development (e.g., congenital adrenal hyperplasia, androgen insensitivity syndrome, Turner syndrome); not a universally accepted term; also called disorders of sex development or intersex
Gender	Societal perception of maleness or femaleness
Genderqueer	Umbrella term for a broad range of identities along or outside the gender continuum; also called gender non-binary
Gender diverse	General term describing gender behaviors, expressions, or identities that are not congruent with those culturally assigned at birth; may include transgender, non-binary, genderqueer, gender fluid, or non–cis-gender identities and may be more dynamic and less stigmatizing than prior terminology (e.g., gender non-forming); this term is not used as a clinical diagnosis
Gender dysphoria	Distress or impairment resulting from incongruence between one's experienced or expressed gender and sex assigned at birth; DSM-5 criteria for adults include at least 6 months of distress or problems functioning due to at least two of the following: • Marked incongruence between one's experienced or expressed gender and primary and/or secondary sex characteristics • Strong desire to be rid of one's primary and/or secondary sex characteristics • Strong desire for the primary and/or secondary sex characteristics of the other gender • Strong desire to be of the other gender • Strong desire to be treated as the other gender • Strong conviction that one has the typical feelings and reactions of the other gender

Table 10.1 (cont.)

Gender expression	External display of gender through appearance (e.g., clothing, hairstyle), behavior, voice, or interests
Gender identity	Internalized sense of self as being male, female, or elsewhere along or outside the gender continuum; some persons have complex identities and may identify as agender, gender non-binary, genderqueer, or gender fluid
Gender identity disorder	Diagnosis related to gender dysphoria or gender incongruence in earlier version of the DSM and ICD
Gender incongruence	General term describing a difference between gender identity and/or expression and designated sex; an ICD-11 diagnosis that does not require a mental health diagnosis
Pansexual	Someone who is attracted to people regardless of their sex or gender identity
Sex	Maleness or femaleness as it relates to sex chromosomes, gonads, genitalia, secondary sex characteristics, and relative levels of sex hormones; these biologic determinants may not necessarily be consistent; sex assigned at birth is typically based on genital anatomy
Sexual orientation	Term describing an enduring physical and emotional attraction to another group; sexual orientation is distinct from gender identity and is self-defined
They/them	Neutral pronouns preferred by some transgendered persons
Transgender	General term used to describe persons whose gender identity or expression differs from their sex assigned at birth
Transgender female	A transgender person designated as male at birth
Transgender male	A transgender person designated as female at birth
Transfeminine	Non-binary term used to describe a feminine spectrum of gender identity
Transmasculine	Non-binary term used to describe a masculine spectrum of gender identity
Transphobia	Prejudicial attitudes about persons who are not cisgender
Transsexual	Historical term, now found offensive by many, for transgender persons seeking medical or surgical therapy to affirm their gender

Because urban environments contain the most densely populated areas in the United States, there is a substantial LGBTQIA+ population in most cities. The multiculturalism and diversity found in many cities is alluring to many LGBTQIA+ people who are searching for a "home away from home" or "chosen family" as they pursue their hopes and dreams. Gay bars were reportedly first opened in the United States in the 1930s, and many of these bars are no longer referred to as "gay bars" because they welcome people from all different backgrounds. The Stonewall Inn, for example, is now a national monument that attracts visitors every day who come to see where the riots took place in 1969. EM providers practicing in urban areas become familiar with taking care of LGBTQIA+ patients.

Gay-Specific Issues

Sexually Transmitted Infections, Pre-Exposure Prophylaxis, and Non-Occupational Post-Exposure Prophylaxis Medications

Many gay men will present to the ED requesting testing, treatment, prophylaxis, and education for sexually transmitted infections (STIs). Common STIs in men include human papillomavirus (HPV), human immunodeficiency virus (HIV), herpes simplex virus (HSV), syphilis, Hepatitis B, Hepatitis C, chlamydia, and gonorrhea.[5] There is also potential for emerging infections, such as Monkeypox. It is important to remember that some of these, specifically HSV, gonorrhea, and chlamydia, may affect a variety of different anatomic locations, including the oropharynx, skin, penis, and/or anus. Some EDs may not have the resources to test for HPV, and the patient should be given outpatient-referral for HPV testing and treatment. It is important to remind gay men that they are more likely to get anal cancer than heterosexual men, and even more so if they have HIV.

Pre-exposure prophylaxis (PrEP) medications are those taken electively and aimed at decreasing one's chances of contracting HIV during sexual encounters or intravenous drug use. Studies show that when taken correctly, PrEP is 99% effective in preventing the spread of HIV. Current regimens of PrEP that are FDA-approved include tenofovir disoproxil and emtriciabine (Truvada), emtricitabine and tenofovir alafenamide (Descovy), and cabotegravir.[6]

Although not an "emergency" *per se*, if a patient presents to the ED with a primary request for PrEP, or requesting PrEP in addition to their primary complaint, it is reasonable for the emergency physician to prescribe it. The patient must be HIV negative, be counseled on the risks and benefits of starting PrEP, and have appropriate follow-up to monitor bloodwork, specifically liver function tests (LFTs) and serum creatinine, and other adverse reactions that may arise while taking PrEP.

By contrast, non-occupational post-exposure prophylaxis medications (nPEP) are taken to minimize the chance of HIV transmission *after* an individual has engaged in sexual intercourse with another individual. An individual may seek the guidance of a healthcare provider if he has had unprotected or partially protected sex or shared an intravenous drug needle with another. They may present to the ED requesting treatment. Ideally, nPEP should begin as soon as possible and within 72 hours of the unprotected encounter. After counseling the patient regarding risks and benefits, the clinician should feel comfortable prescribing nPEP for them. One common regimen includes a 28-day course of emtricitabine/tenofovir. While screening patients for nPEP, patients should have other tests performed as well. HIV, Hepatitis B/C, syphilis, gonorrhea, pregnancy (when appropriate), serum creatinine, and serum LFTs should be checked. Clinicians should then ensure that their patients have proper follow-up for repeat testing.[7]

Recreational Drug Use

Recreational drug use and prescription drug misuse are disproportionately present in the urban LGBTQIA+ community. According to the Substance Abuse and Mental Health Services Administration's 2015 National Survey on Drug Use and Mental Health, 39% of sexual minorities (defined as lesbian, gay, or bisexual for the purposes of this survey) admitted to having used an illicit drug in the previous year, compared to 17% of the sexual majority. In this survey, the sexual minorities were more likely to have used marijuana, cocaine, hallucinogens, methamphetamines, inhalants, and heroin. They were also more likely to misuse prescription drugs for recreational purposes.[8]

Some gay men participate in chemsex, which is the "use of drugs before or during planned sexual events to facilitate, enhance, prolong, and sustain the experience."[8] Such drugs may include methamphetamines, cocaine, gamma hydroxybutyrate (GHB), ketamine, and others. Some gay men may come into the ED, reporting that they have used one or many of these drugs during a sexual experience. Events that may provide opportunities for chemsex include sex parties, raves, or circuit parties, which are large gay parties that can include drugs and dancing. Some gay men may unintentionally or unknowingly take drugs, so if partners or companions are present, they may provide valuable collateral information, especially if the patient is comatose or otherwise unable to participate in interview.[9]

Some gay men may present to the ED with complaints related to anabolic androgen steroid (AAS) use. In one study, it was found that 21.6% of gay and bisexual men have used AAS in their lifetime.[10] AAS have many adverse side effects, including hypertension, cardiomyopathy, thromboembolism, arrhythmias, coronary artery disease, cholestasis, mood disorders, and aggression.[11,12] It is not uncommon for men to conceal their use of AAS (as some are illegal), so patients should be reassured that any disclosures of this nature are confidential. Also, many AAS are administered using needles, so infections can be spread this way as well.

Lesbian-Specific Issues

Pregnancy Testing

The indications for and appropriateness of pregnancy testing in lesbian patients should be considered in every clinical encounter. If a lesbian patient is only sexually active with other lesbians and has not been attempting to become pregnant via insemination or in-vitro fertilization, she may eschew a clinician-recommended pregnancy test. Others may accept them because they feel it is the path of least resistance. Most radiology departments require that women of child-bearing age undergo a pregnancy test prior to radiographic imaging, but many offer a waiver to be signed if the patient does not want to submit to testing. It is important to utilize joint decision making with the patient, taking into consideration her risk of pregnancy, the implications of a missed pregnancy (for instance, if the chief complaint is abdominal pain and vaginal bleeding). Ultimately, shared decision making should always be used in these circumstances.

Pelvic Exam

Special consideration should be given to lesbian patients when a pelvic exam is deemed necessary. Many have never had penetrative vaginal intercourse, and if they have never been examined by an obstetrician-gynecologist they may not be accustomed to or comfortable with a pelvic exam. The clinician should be particularly sensitive to these considerations when determining the need for the exam and the manner in which it is to be performed.

Sexually Transmitted Infections

Sexually transmitted infections are important to consider in women who have sex with women. Sexual adjuncts, such as vibrators, are capable of transmitting STIs, and may do so even after cleaning.[13,14] It may be important to inquire about use of such adjuncts when taking a sexual history, and counsel patients accordingly. Additional counseling may relate to the fact that some STIs, including Hepatitis C, are more common in women who have sex with women. Similarly, although not always considered an STI, bacterial vaginosis was also more common in lesbians.[15]

Transgender-Specific Issues

Transgender people encompass a diverse group but share the commonality that their gender expression or identity is different from the gender they were assigned at birth. Some transgender people choose to have gender affirmation surgery, and others do not. Gender affirmation surgery can include facial surgery, top surgery, or bottom surgery. Female to male top surgery is a procedure that aims to remove excess fat and skin in order to create a natural-appearing flat chest. Bottom surgery involves transforming genitalia for the patient to match their gender expression and/or identity. Many patients may have the desire to have gender affirmation surgery (which may include several procedures) but have not begun or are just beginning the process. It is important to note that many of the surgeries have complications and the patients may form close relationships with their gender affirmation surgeons, but when unavailable, general and/or plastic surgery consultants may be utilized to help guide decision-making.[16]

In addition to surgical procedures, transgender patients may be on a variety of medications. Transgender women may decide to take estrogen, and transgender men may decide to take testosterone. In one study, 67%–78% of transgender women were taking hormones for gender affirmation.[17] There are many different routes and formulations the transgender patient may decide to take, so the provider should be cognizant of asking the exact medication and dosage. Taking exogenous hormones may increase the transgender patient's risk of cardiovascular events. It is important to note that pediatric patients may have already begun taking hormone therapy, and that some patients may have started taking hormone therapy on their own without the guidance of a physician. In such circumstances, the patient should be dissuaded from doing so. Furthermore, when making clinical decisions and forming lists of differential diagnoses, clinicians should remember that any patient with a uterus may become pregnant.

It is important to note that the clinician must always try to make the transgender patient feel comfortable. When genitourinary or rectal exams are necessary, the sex of the chaperone should match the gender identity of the patient and institutional policy should reflect this and should adhere to institutional policies. The transgender patient also may refer to their genitals with different words than the terms assigned to their genitalia at birth. For example, a transgender male who has a vagina may refer to it as his "front hole." If the clinician inadvertently makes a mistake of terminology, an acknowledgment and apology is advised.

Bisexual, Pansexual, and "Discreet" Patients

Many patients may present to the ED stating that they have engaged in sexual acts with a partner who may not be their typical or always-preferred sexual preference. Some people consider themselves "discreet" (formerly described colloquially as the "down-low" population), which can mean that they live an outwardly heterosexual life but have sex with members of the homosexual, transgender, or other communities in a clandestine fashion. These patients should be supported and encouraged to be forthcoming regarding all sexual partners so that STI risk can be understood and all partners can be appropriately addressed.

Pansexual persons feel attraction regardless of gender and may have sex with people of any gender identity or expressions. Other people may not consider themselves homosexual, yet they have sex with the same sex in the context of legal or illegal entertainment or sex work, or may simply be questioning or experimenting with their sexuality.

LGBTQIA+ Youth

Compared to heterosexual teens, LGBTQIA+ youth are more likely to attempt suicide, to experience physical dating violence, electronic/physical bullying, and forced sexual intercourse. Of LGBTQIA+ youth, 30.5% reported persistent feelings of sadness and hopelessness. LGBTQIA+ are also more likely to abuse alcohol, marijuana, and prescription opioids and are also more likely to have a higher lifetime risk of abusing other drugs as well, including other drugs such as cocaine, methamphetamines, heroin, and other drugs of abuse.[18,19] A parent may or may not accompany their LGBTQIA+ child to the ED. If the minor patient is accompanied by a parent, it is prudent to ask to speak to the patient alone regarding their social history, which can include questions on drugs, sex, sexual orientation, communicable disease, etc. Once the provider has finished asking the minor questions about their social history, it may be appropriate to ask the minor if they would like help talking to their parent about sensitive issues.

Mental Health

There are mental health considerations when treating LGBTQIA+ patients. One meta-analysis of 25 studies found that LGBTQIA+ adults and children over age 12 also had a two-fold increased risk of suicide attempts and were 1.5 times more likely to have depression and anxiety.[20]

It is important for clinicians to ask LGBTQIA+ patients if they are experiencing any form of abuse from their partner(s). Besides physical and sexual forms of abuse, there are many other types of abuse , which can include one partner threatening to "out" the other, or one partner forcing the other to hide their sexuality. Clinicians may not be as attuned to same-sex partner abuse, as they may incorrectly perceive "masculine" individuals as able to defend themselves, or may not ask female patients in same-sex relationships if they feel threatened or unsafe in their relationship.[21]

LGBTQIA+ Empowerment

Many healthcare providers consider themselves to be part of the LGBTQIA+ community. Some share their sexuality or gender expression/identity and some do not. Similar to a heterosexual provider referencing their "wife" or "husband" during a conversation with a patient, an LGBTQIA+ provider may feel comfortable doing the same. Or they may elect to reference their significant other as their "partner". LGBTQIA+ clinicians may feel comfortable discussing their experiences with LGBTQIA+ sports leagues, choirs, musicals, drag shows, queer parties, adoption, surrogacy, in-vitro fertilization, career counselors, LGBTQIA+ friends, family, and many other topics. Regardless, no one should be questioned about or expected to disclose or elucidate any of the above information beyond what they volunteer in the workplace.

Some additional resources are provided in Table 10.2.

Table 10.2 Some Additional Resources That Providers, Support Staff, and Patients May Find Helpful

Trans Lifeline: Crisis/Suicide hotline for Transgender individuals (www.translifeline.org) 877-565-8860

Trevor Project: Crisis/Suicide Hotline for LGBT Teens (www.thetrevorproject.org) 1-866-488-7386

World Professional Association for Transgender Health: health organization focusing on treatment and education of gender dysphoria (www.wpath.org)

Gay, Lesbian, and Straight Education Network: Education network focusing on anti-bullying of students who are sexual and gender minorities (www.glsen.org)

Gay, Lesbian, and Straight Education Network: Education network focusing on anti-bullying of students who are sexual and gender minorities (www.glsen.org)

YES Institute: Their mission is to prevent suicide and ensure the healthy development of all youth through powerful communication and education on gender and orientation; based in Miami Florida (https://yesinstitute.org)

Gender Spectrum: https://genderspectrum.org/

PFLAG: https://pflag.org/about

Trans Student Educational Resources: https://transstudent.org/

Family Acceptance Project https://familyproject.sfsu.edu/

Vignette Conclusion

The provider immediately goes to meet the patient before she leaves. He introduces himself and asks her preferred name and gender identity. He sincerely apologizes for the way she was treated by the hospital staff and ensures her that it is unacceptable that she was treated this way. He reiterates that he wants to help her and will take her to a private room with a nurse and conducts a thorough history and physical examination. He also informs her that he will help her make a formal complaint with patient relations regarding the discrimination she experienced if she chooses to do so.

Pro-Tips

- Develop a working familiarity with gender-related terminology so as to understand patient-specific needs and create a trusting and mutually respectful rapport with patients.
- Maintain awareness and appreciation of the medical and psychosocial needs of LGBTQIA + patients.
- Be diligent in maintaining the particular privacy concerns of LBBTQIA+ youth.

References

1. Sue DW. *Microaggressions in Everyday Life: Race, Gender, and Sexual Orientation*. John Wiley & Sons, 2010.

2. Dean, MA, Victor E, Guidry-Grimes L. Inhospitable healthcare spaces. Why diversity training on LGBTQIA patients is not enough. *J Bioethical Inq,* 2016;13:557–570.

3. Moll J, Krieger P, Heron SL, Joyce C, Moreno-Walton L. Attitudes, behavior, and

comfort of emergency medicine residents in caring for LGBT patients: what do we know? *AEM Educ Train.* 2019; (2):129–135.

4. Govere L, Govere EM. How effective is cultural competence training of healthcare providers on improving patient satisfaction of minority groups? A systematic review of literature. *Worldviews Evid-Based Nurs.* 2016;13(6):402–410.

5. Center for Disease Control and Prevention. Gay and bisexual men's health: sexually transmitted diseases. 2016. www.cdc.gov/ msmhealth/STD.htm

6. Center for Disease Control and Prevention. Updated guidelines for antiretroviral postexposure prophylaxis after sexual, injection drug use, or other nonoccupational exposure to HIV – United States. 2016, updated 2018. https://stacks.cdc.gov/view/cdc/38856

7. Substance Abuse and Mental Health Services Administration. Sexual orientation and estimates of adult substance use and mental health: results from the 2015 National Survey on Drug Use and Health. 2015. www.samhsa.gov/data/sites/default/fi les/NSDUH-SexualOrientation-2015/NSD UH-SexualOrientation-2015/NSDUH-SexualOrientation-2015.htm

8. Maxwell S, Shahmanesh M, Gafos M. Chemsex behaviours among men who have sex with men: a systematic review of the literature. *Int J Drug Policy.* 2019;63:74–89. doi: 10.1016/j.drugpo.2018.11.014. PMID: 30513473.

9. Ip E, Doroudgar S, Shah-Manek B, Barnett MJ, Tenerowicz MJ, Ortanez M, Pope Jr HG. The CASTRO study: unsafe sexual behaviors and illicit drug use among gay and bisexual men who use anabolic steroids. *Am J Addict.* 2019;28 (2):101.

10. Liu J-D, Wu Y-Q. Anabolic-androgenic steroids and cardiovascular risk. *Chinese Med J.* 2019;132(18):2229–2236.

11. Albano GD, Amico F, Cocimano G, Liberto A, Maglietta F, Esposito M, Li

Rosi G, Di Nunno N, Salerno M, Montana A. Adverse effects of anabolic-androgenic steroids: a literature review. *Healthcare (Basel).* 2021;9(1):97.

12. Frimpon E, Rowan GA, Williams D, Li M, Solano L, Chaudhry S, Radigan M. Health disparities, inpatient stays, and emergency room visits among lesbian, gay, and bisexual people: evidence from a mental health system.*Psychiatr Serv.* 2020;71:128–135.

13. Anderson TA, Schick V, Herbenik D, Dodge B, Fortenberry JD. A study of human papillomavirus on vaginally inserted sex toys, before and after cleaning, among women who have sex with women and men. *Sex Transm Infect.* 2014;90:529–531.

14. Fethers K, Marks C, Mindel A, Estcourt CS. Sexually transmitted infections and risk behaviours in women who have sex with women. *Sex Transm Infect.* 2000;76:345–349.

15. The Cleveland Clinic. Gender affirmation (confirmation) or sex reassignment surgery. 2021. https://my.clevelandclinic.org/health/ treatments/21526-gender-affirmation-confirmation-or-sex-reassignment-surgery

16. Center for Disease Control and Prevention. HIV infection, risk, prevention, and testing behaviors among transgender women: National HIV Behavioral Surveillance 7 U.S. Cities, 2019–2020. 2021. www.cdc.gov /hiv/pdf/library/reports/surveillance/cdc-hiv-surveillance-special-report-number-27 .pdf

17. Unger CA. Hormone therapy for transgender patients. *Transl Androl Urol.* 2016;5(6):877–884.

18. Center for Disease Control and Prevention. Youth Risk Behavior Surveillance (YRBS). 2020. www.cdc.gov/healthyyouth/data/yrb s/index.htm

19. Center for Disease Control and Prevention. Youth Risk Behavior Surveillance – United States, 2019. *MMWR.* 2020;69(1). www .cdc.gov/mmwr/volumes/69/su/pdfs/s u6901-H.pdf

20. King M, Semlyen J, Tai SS, Killaspy H, Osborn D, Popelyuk D, Nazareth IA. Systematic review of mental disorder, suicide, and deliberate self harm in lesbian, gay and bisexual people. *BMC Psychiatry*. 2008;18;8:70.

21. Bermea AM, Slakoff DC, Goldberg AE. Intimate partner violence in the LGBTQ+ community: experiences, outcomes, and implications for primary care. *Prim Care*. 2021;48 (2):329–337.

Child Maltreatment

Nisha Narayanan and Dana Lauture

11

Vignette

A 6-week-old previously healthy male child, born full-term via a normal spontaneous vaginal delivery, presents to your emergency department (ED) with his mother with a bump on the back of his head. The mother states that she was changing his diaper 3 days prior when the patient rolled off his changing table and fell from about 3 feet onto a hardwood floor. He cried immediately and had no loss of consciousness, vomiting, or seizure activity. He has been crying "a little more than normal" since his injury but remains consolable. He is waking up to feed every 3 hours and is urinating and stooling normally. Mom brought him to the ED because the lump has persisted for 3 days and "isn't getting smaller." The patient lives with his 15-year-old mom and maternal grandmother only. Dad is not involved in the child's care.

Vital signs are stable, and the patient appears well. There is a 3-cm hematoma on the baby's parietal scalp and the base can be palpated. The rest of his exam is unremarkable albeit limited as he is drinking formula comfortably throughout the exam and the mother requests that you return the child. Brief examination over his "onesie" reveals that heart and lung are normal, abdomen is soft, and there are no notable areas of tenderness on exam.

- What is the next step in managing this patient?
- What are this child's risk factors for child abuse?
- Are there any "red flags" in this child's history that would raise suspicion for child abuse?

Introduction

Child maltreatment encompasses both abuse and neglect. The Federal Child Abuse Prevention and Treatment Act defines child abuse and neglect as "any recent act or failure to act on the part of a parent or caretaker, which results in the death, serious physical or emotional harm, sexual abuse, or exploitation of a child or an act or failure to act which presents an imminent risk of serious harm." A "child" under this definition generally means a person who is younger than age 18 or who is not an emancipated minor.

Child maltreatment can be divided into seven main categories: physical abuse, sexual abuse, emotional abuse, physical neglect, emotional neglect, medical neglect, and educational neglect.[1,2] These specific definitions vary among the different states and institutions; however, the general principles are consistent nationally (Table 11.1).

Child abuse is a global problem. Data from many low- and middle-income countries are lacking, thus numbers are underreported.[4] In addition, many deaths due to child maltreatment are attributed to drowning, falls, and other unintentional injuries. Per World Health

Table 11.1 Categories of Child Maltreatment

Keyword	Definition
Physical abuse	The intentional use of physical force that can result in physical injury. Examples include hitting, kicking, shaking, burning, or other shows of force against a child[1]
Sexual abuse	Pressuring or forcing a child to engage in sexual acts. It includes behaviors such as fondling, penetration, and exposing a child to other sexual activities[1]
Emotional abuse	Behaviors that harm a child's self-worth or emotional well-being. Examples include name-calling, shaming, rejection, withholding love, and threatening[2]
Physical neglect	The failure of a parent or caretaker to meet the child's basic physical needs such as food, clothing, or shelter. It often occurs in a persistent pattern. Examples include being denied food, leaving the child with an impaired caregiver, or leaving a child out in the cold
Emotional neglect	Inattention to the child's need for affection, and the refusal of or failure to provide needed psychological care. Also includes spousal abuse in the presence of the child and permission to use drugs or alcohol by the child[3]
Medical neglect	The failure to provide a child with necessary medical, dental, or in some cases mental health care. An example is delaying immediate medical care after a child clearly fractures their arm
Educational neglect	Failure to support a child's educational needs either by keeping a child home from school for unexcused reasons or not following up with a child's educational needs despite the school's outreach to the parent or caretaker[1]

Organization data, nearly 3 in 4 children or 300 million children aged 2–4 years regularly suffer physical punishment and/or psychological violence at the hands of parents and caregivers. One in five women and 1 in 13 men report having been sexually abused as a child. One hundred and twenty million girls and young women under 20 years of age have additionally suffered some form of forced sexual contact.

In the United States alone, the Centers for Disease Control and Prevention cite that at least 1 in 7 children have experienced child maltreatment in the past year, and this is likely an underestimate. In 2020, 1750 children died of abuse and neglect nationally, making it a significant cause of pediatric morbidity and mortality and the third leading cause of death in children between one and four years of age.[4] Of note, increases in child maltreatment have been well-documented during and after recessions and epidemics when parental stressors are high and there is a loss of financial and social supports. The most common type of abuse of which the urban practitioner should be aware is physical abuse followed by emotional abuse, then sexual abuse. The most common form of neglect is physical neglect.[5]

The consequences of child maltreatment include impaired lifelong physical and mental health. A child who is abused is more likely to abuse others as an adult, thus the cycle of violence persists, and it is critical to break. Maltreatment causes stress that is associated with disruption of early brain development, and extreme stress can impair nervous and immune system development. Maltreated children are also at increased risk for behavioral, physical, and mental health problems in adulthood such as depression, obesity, smoking, being the victim of perpetrator of violence, not graduating from school, unintended pregnancy, alcohol, and drug misuse.[4]

Findings are mixed on whether rates of child maltreatment are higher in urban or rural areas. Several sources have shown that the prevalence of child maltreatment is similar across the urban–rural spectrum,[6] while others have demonstrated that children living in rural communities are more likely to experience abuse.[5] Some reports show that the risk factors for child abuse vary among urban and rural areas. Regardless, the poverty, community violence, and high population density in metropolitan areas ensures that the average urban practitioner will encounter numerous suspected abuse cases and must develop the skills to adequately identify and address them.

What certainly differs among urban and rural settings are disparities in ED management. Urban EDs have more community programs in place to help at-risk families, more resources to help children who are being maltreated, and are also more likely to have a child abuse expert on site or easily available. The urban practitioner must learn to recognize the patients who will benefit from such interventions to promote the health and well-being of the entire community and break the cycle of child abuse and neglect. We introduce a systematic approach to identifying and managing a child with abuse who presents to the urban ED, first explaining each step and then uniting the steps into a sequential framework.

Risk Factors for Abuse

There are multiple characteristics, or risk factors, that may increase the likelihood that a child in an urban environment may experience maltreatment. They must be kept in mind with each patient but cautiously employed to avoid bias. These factors can be divided into characteristics of the individual child, the caregiver, the family, and the community but they are all interrelated and additive (Figure 11.1).

Individual Risk Factors

At-risk children include those who are younger than four years of age and adolescents, and those with special needs who may increase the caregiver burden (emotional/behavioral difficulties, special needs, chronic illness, physical disabilities, developmental disabilities, or

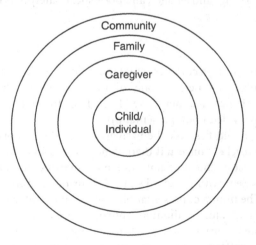

Figure 11.1 Risk factors for child abuse in an urban environment

neurological disorders). Other risk factors include being born prematurely, being an unwanted child, and being the result of an unplanned pregnancy. Children identifying as or being identified as lesbian, gay, bisexual, or transgender are at risk as well.[7]

Caregiver Risk Factors

Caregiver risk factors associated with higher rates of child abuse include caregivers with depression or other mental illness, low self-esteem, poor impulse control, substance abuse/alcohol abuse, young maternal or paternal age, low education level, low income or unemployment, and having poor knowledge of child development or unrealistic expectations for a child. History of caregiver abuse or neglect as a child, high levels of caregiver stress, and single parents or parents with many children are also risk factors. In addition, having caregivers in the home who are not a biological parent or a caregiver who uses spanking or other forms or corporal punishment for discipline increases a child's risk for maltreatment.[7]

Family Risk Factors

Children in families with household members in prison, high conflict and negative communication styles, and those who experience social isolation (not connected to neighbors, extended family, or friends) are at risk for maltreatment. Families experiencing or who have experienced other types of violence such as domestic violence place children at increased risk as well.[8]

Community Risk Factors

The living environment of the child and the social norms to which they are exposed greatly affect their risk of maltreatment. Communities with high rates of crime and violence, high rates of poverty, limited educational and economic opportunities, high rates of unemployment, food insecurity, unstable housing, few community activities, and low rates of community involvement where neighbors do not know each other have similarly high rates of child maltreatment. In addition, communities that have poor or non-enforced child protection laws, easy access to drugs and alcohol, and poor social safety nets have increased rates of child abuse.[7,8]

Clinical History

As with any patient encounter, a complete child maltreatment–focused history should begin with the history of present illness. Details of the story should be obtained in a non-accusatory and chronological manner. Several red flags for child abuse can be identified solely on the history provided upon presentation.

The ED clinician should first ask themselves, "Does this history make sense?" There should be an elevated level of concern if there is no explanation or a vague explanation for a significant injury. A history that does not explain the injuries identified or one in which the explanation is inconsistent with the child's physical or developmental ability should raise suspicion for abuse. The timing of presentation is also important; a notable delay in seeking medical attention for any injury without an appropriate reason is concerning. So too is an important detail of the history changing significantly over time or an explanation that is inconsistent with the pattern, age, or severity of the injury (see Table 11.2). Different

Table 11.2 Historical Components That May Suggest Intentional Trauma[9]

No explanation/vague explanation for a significant injury
History or important detail of history changes over time
History does not explain injury identified
History is inconsistent with the age of injury
Notable delay in seeking medical care
Explanation is inconsistent with child's physical ability
Explanation is inconsistent with child's developmental ability
Explanation is inconsistent with the pattern or severity of the injury

witnesses providing markedly different explanations for the injury warrant additional investigation. Interactions between the child and the parent and between the child and clinical staff members are also helpful to note.[7]

A thorough review of systems should be performed next, followed by obtaining the past medical history, which should include chronic illnesses, congenital disorders, prior history of trauma and previous hospitalizations, and details about the pregnancy and birth history.

A detailed social history should be obtained. A list of everyone living in the home with the child should be included, along with any non-family household members. It should be noted if there is a history of substance abuse or violent interactions among any of those household members, the methods of discipline, and any open Child Protective Services (CPS) cases. Age-specific school questions such as school performance and attendance should be posed, as should questions about recent family stressors and financial issues. The child should also be interviewed alone if this is age-appropriate. Open-ended and non-leading questions should be asked in a neutral tone. Questions and answers should be recorded verbatim.

When taking a family history in a child with suspected child maltreatment, clinicians must inquire about the presence of any significant genetic, metabolic, bone, bleeding, or skin disorders in the family. There are organic medical conditions that may be confused with physical or sexual abuse (see Table 11.3), which must be considered. A patient who comes in with multiple fractures in different ages of healing, for example, may in fact have an underlying genetic disease such as osteogenesis imperfecta, but could be mistaken for being a victim of child abuse.[10]

The Physical Exam

In addition to the usual components of a physical exam, the patient's height, weight, and head circumference should be plotted on a growth chart, to ensure that growth velocity has been appropriate. A thorough head to toe exam should be performed in all cases concerning for child maltreatment. The genital exam should be included, especially when there is a concern for sexual abuse. Injuries should be evaluated objectively and documented in detail.

As with the history, red flags for child abuse may also be identified on physical exam (Table 11.4). Clinicians should look for head injuries, signs of abdominal injuries, patterned burns, bruises, and specific types of fractures. Sentinel injuries are defined as visible, minor, poorly explained injuries in young infants that are concerning for abuse.[11] Often times,

Table 11.3 Physical findings that may be confused for abuse and possible alternative causes

Bruising	Dermal melanocystosis Vasculitis (i.e., IgA vasculitis) Hemangioma Ehlers–Danlos syndrome Menkes disease Bleeding disorders (i.e., hemophilia) Idiopathic thrombocytic purpura Leukemia
Intracranial bleed/abusive head trauma	Hemorrhagic disease of the newborn (vitamin K deficiency) Glutaric aciduria type 1 (macrocranium, subdural hematoma, sparse intraretinal and preretinal hemorrhages, and frontotemporal atrophy) Birth trauma or accidental trauma Infection Vascular anomalies (hemangioma, AV malformation)
Fractures	Osteogenesis imperfecta Neuromuscular disorders Osteopenia secondary to limited mobility in children with cerebral palsy Rickets Neoplasm Vitamin C deficiency Ehlers–Danlos syndrome Menkes disease
Burns	Phytophotodermatitis Impetigo *Staphylococcus*-mediated disease (i.e., *Staphylococcus*-scalded skin syndrome, bullous impetigo)
Other patterned skin findings	Cupping, coining, spooning (and other alternative and complementary medicine therapies)
Sexual abuse	Lichen sclerosis Lichen planus Anal fissures from constipation or straining Labial adhesions Bechet's disease Chrohn's disease Psoriasis Eczema Molluscum contagiosum

infants present multiple times with different sentinel injuries before they are evaluated for abuse, thus a thorough exam is essential. Sentinel injuries may include skin findings such as bruises, oral injuries such as torn frenulum, or ocular findings such as subconjunctival and retinal hemorrhages.[11]

Table 11.4 Exam Components of a Complete Exam to Evaluate for Child Maltreatment[12,13]

Exam component	Possible abnormal finding/cause
General assessment of alertness, eye opening, and responsiveness	Intracranial hemorrhage, head injury
Height, weight, head circumference (compared with past measurements, if possible)	Failure to thrive, neglect, or growth failure
Mouth and teeth examination	Dental caries suggestive of neglect Torn labial frenulum suggestive of abuse Broken teeth/mouth injury
Scalp examination	Patchy hair loss caused by traumatic alopecia or severe malnutrition
Funduscopic examination of the eyes	Retinal hemorrhages
Skin examination for bruising	Multiple patterns of bruising suggestive of abuse • Bruise in child younger than 4 months • Bruise in torso, ear, and neck areas • Ear bruising (suggests "boxing ears") • Buttocks bruising • Bite marks • Patterned bruises (hand, cord, belt, object) Bruises at different stages of healing
Skin examination for burns	Multiple burns of varying ages and types Specific patterned burn injuries • Buttock and lower leg burns or hand burns with a sharp demarcation between burned and normal skin and sparing of flexed protected areas (suggests immersion injury) • round, small, punched out burns (suggests cigarette burn) • contact burns in clear shape of a hot object (e.g., curling iron, fork, cigarette lighter, clothing iron)
Palpation for tenderness or bony bumps/irregularities, especially of the neck, torso, and extremities	Occult fracture, past fracture if callus can be palpated
Finger and nail examination	Dirty nails suggestive of neglect Broken fingers or nails suggestive of abuse
Genital exam	Anal tears or genital injury suggestive of recent abuse*
Deep tendon reflexes, muscle tone, or responsiveness to tactile stimuli	Spinal cord injury

* Even in the presence of sexual abuse, most genital exams are normal.

Head injuries from non-accidental trauma tend to result in more significant pathology than from accidental trauma.[13] Abusive head trauma is the inflicted head injury of a child that can involve a variety of biomechanical forces, including shaking. It is fatal in nearly a quarter of cases.[14] Shaking a baby violently can cause subdural hematomas, subarachnoid hemorrhages, and direct trauma to the brain matter itself if there is sudden deceleration of the head when it impacts a surface. Clinical manifestations may be subtle, and may only include fussiness or mild vomiting. You may see scalp hematomas or scalp lacerations. There may not be focal neurological deficits on neurological exam. Infants may be irritable or lethargic in severe cases. An ophthalmologic exam with fundoscopy must be performed to assess for the presence of retinal hemorrhages, which would be highly suspicious for abusive head trauma.[15] The amount of retinal hemorrhages seen correlates with the degree of intracranial injury.[13]

In infants, oral injuries such as a torn frenulum from forceful feeding is a classic sign of physical abuse. Torn frenulums, however, can result from accidental mechanisms as well and are NOT pathognomonic for child abuse.

Injuries to the chest may involve squeezing of the thorax or blunt trauma, which may result in rib fractures or bruising on the thorax. Rib fractures, especially those located posterolaterally, are highly suggestive of abuse. A caregiver may report a false story of providing chest compressions. Abdominal injuries may involve either solid and/or viscus organs. These injuries should be considered if abdominal exam is positive for abdominal tenderness or guarding.[13]

Other signs of abuse include fractures caused by a twisting or pulling mechanism. Fractures involving the ribs, scapula, or sternum are also suspicious. Palpation of the bones of the extremities, ribs, and skull should be performed. Callus formation may occur in older fractures that are in the healing stages and may be felt during the exam.

Although accidental injuries often occur on bony prominences, inflicted injuries tend to occur in protected areas, such as the neck, buttocks, trunk, and upper arms.[6] The TEN-4 bruising clinical decision rule may be useful to identify children and infants who should be evaluated for physical abuse.[16] It states that bruising on the torso, ear, or neck (TEN) in a child 4 years or younger, or bruising of any region in a child younger than 4 months, requires further evaluation for abuse. The initial study of 95 children younger than 48 months who were admitted to a pediatric intensive care unit because of trauma reported a sensitivity and specificity of 97% and 84%, respectively.[17]

Bruises on extremities with a logical explanation, even if they are numerous and are in various stages of healing, are common as children get minor injuries all the time. Bruises located centrally (torso, ear, neck) are more concerning for abuse, especially in infants who are not yet ambulatory. Bruises seen in babies less than 6 months old are often due to abuse. Remember – "if they don't cruise, they don't bruise."

A genital exam should be performed in all cases of suspected child maltreatment. The majority of child victims of sexual abuse will have a normal physical exam.[18] Injuries in the genital area often heal without any notable abnormalities. Many forms of sexual abuse do not cause physical injury, and many sexual abuse victims do not seek medical care until long after the abuse. Many physical findings that may appear abnormal are just normal variants. The exam should be performed in a way that minimizes the patient's anxiety. Boys may be examined in a sitting, supine, or standing position and the penis, testicles, and perineum should be examined. Practitioners should position girls in a non-invasive and non-painful manner such as in a supine frog-leg position with their knees apart. The child can sit on their caregiver for the examination in this position. They can alternatively sit in a prone, knee to chest position with their head and chest on the exam table. Girls may spread their own labia if they prefer. No speculum exam or digital penetration should be employed in pre-pubertal girls unless there is active genital bleeding; in this case, sedation may be necessary. Locations of abnormalities should be described using a clock face; the urethra is the 12 o'clock position and the anus is the 6 o'clock position. In both boys and girls, an external anus exam should be performed with gentle retraction of the gluteal folds.[14]

Urban medical settings typically have nearby child advocacy centers, which include social services, law enforcement agencies, legal services, and specialized medical and forensic evaluation. The advocacy center can be a resource for consultation or for a more thorough genital exam if this is necessary; however, the basic external exam should still be performed in the ED. If a sexual assault has occurred within 96 hours of the ED visit, the patient or caregiver may choose to have forensic evidence collected via a specialized forensic exam in case charges will be pursued. Some centers are fortunate to have certified Sexual Assault Forensics Examiners (SAFE) who can perform the exam; however, pediatric-trained SAFE examiners are rare and thus the responsibility often falls on the shoulders of the emergency medicine physician. Given that the exam is somewhat invasive, involving the child protection team in this process and asking for advice is helpful.

After the physical examination, discuss and document your findings. Skin findings should be well-described, including the location, measurements, and shapes. All dermatologic conditions (eczema, psoriasis) as well as bruising, trauma, etc. should be included. Burns that have an obvious pattern to them such as a submersion pattern, cigarette burn patterns, or patterns that resemble any object used to burn the child should be specifically noted. Photographs should be obtained whenever possible and uploaded into the patient's chart.

Organic medical conditions may be confused with physical or sexual abuse (Table 11.4). Coagulopathies and bleeding disorders may mimic trauma. Rickets and osteogenesis imperfecta may result in easy fractures. Conditions that may mimic abusive head trauma include hemorrhagic disease of the newborn, which may be especially common in neonates who were born at home and never received a vitamin K injection at birth. There are also numerous cutaneous findings that may be confused for abuse, such as hemangiomas and dermal melanocytosis. It is important for urban clinicians to consider these conditions while evaluating every suspected case of child maltreatment.

Laboratory Studies and Imaging

Children with suspected abuse require further evaluation for two purposes: to identify medical disorders that may explain observed findings and to search for more severe injury than may be evident on initial exam. Routine testing in such patients includes blood work and imaging.

Laboratory screening should include a complete blood count (CBC), a basic metabolic panel, liver function tests, amylase and lipase, coagulation studies, urinalysis, and urine toxicology. Hepatic transaminase levels have a modest sensitivity and specificity (77% and 82%, respectively) for occult abdominal injuries at a cutoff level of 80 U per liter.[16] Depending on the patient's presentation, additional electrolyte, hormone, and factor levels, urine toxicology, and other bleeding studies may be ordered as well (see Table 11.3). The decision to perform sexually transmitted infection testing is made on a case-by-case basis[19] (Table 11.5).

Table 11.5 Laboratory Testing in the Child With Suspected Maltreatment[13]

Test	Reason for test
CBC, coagulation factors (PT/PTT/INR)	Rule out coagulopathy/bleeding disorder causing unexplained bruising or bleeding
AST, ALT, amylase, lipase levels	Rule out occult abdominal injury
BMP, urinalysis	Rule out occult renal injury
Toxicology screen	Rule out poisoning or overdose
Calcium, alkaline phosphatase, phosphorus, albumin, parathyroid hormone levels	Rule out malnutrition, bone mineralization disorders (e.g., rickets)
Fibrinogen, von Willebrand factor, platelet aggregation studies, clotting factor assays	Rule out coagulopathy causing unexplained bruising or bleeding

Appropriate imaging studies are essential to rule out occult injury in the evaluation and management of child abuse, particularly in the small child who is unable to communicate.

All children less than 2 years old with suspected abuse or children with difficulty communicating should undergo a skeletal survey. A skeletal survey is a series of radiographs, performed systematically to cover the entire skeleton. It aims to accurately identify abnormalities and differentiate them from developmental changes and other anatomic variants that may occur in infants. A typical skeletal survey includes bilateral anteroposterior (AP) and posteroanterior (PA) projections of hands, forearms, humerus, thorax, forearms, feet, lower legs, femur, pelvis, spine, and skull. A joint survey includes bilateral AP and PA views of wrist, elbow, shoulder, ankle, knee, hip, and sacroiliac joints. The skeletal survey differs from a "babygram," or a single, non-targeted radiograph of an infant, which is insufficient.

In children 2–5 years old, the decision to image is guided by other findings of possible abuse and is performed in cases where abuse is strongly suspected. In children older than 5 years, imaging should be based on clinical findings and children can usually give a sufficient history of pain. Each area of interest should thus be imaged separately.

A non-contrast computed tomography (CT) or magnetic resonance imaging (MRI) of the head should be considered in all children with suspected abuse to evaluate for abusive head trauma. It is a mandatory test in children less than 6 months old, although its urgency is up for debate. In addition, abdominal ultrasounds and MRIs should be considered in all cases with suspected intra-abdominal injury.

There are several imaging findings that are specific for child abuse. Highly specific injuries include classic metaphyseal lesions, also known as corner fractures or "bucket handle fractures," posterolateral rib fractures, and any fractures involving the sternum, scapula, or spinous processes (Figures 11.2–11.5). Moderately specific injuries include multiple fractures, fractures in various stages of healing, epiphyseal separation, vertebral body fractures and subluxations, digital fractures, and complex skull fractures. Less specific for abuse include clavicular fractures, as these are common fractures. Spiral fractures are the result of a forceful twisting or jerking of an extremity. They are common in preschool children and toddlers who can walk; however, they are suspicious for abuse in very young immobile children.

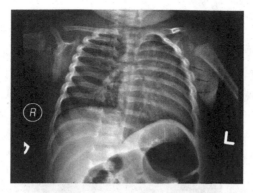

Figure 11.2 Non-displaced right scapular spine fracture and multiple left-sided rib fractures in stages of healing. Image used with permission from VisualDx (www.visualdx.com)

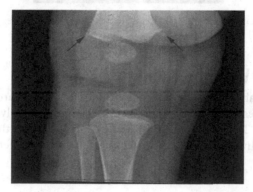

Figure 11.3 Metaphyseal corner fractures of the medial and lateral aspects of the distal femur. Images used with permission from VisualDx (www.visualdx.com)

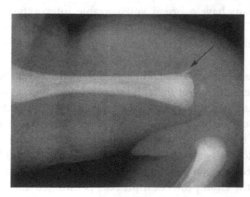

Figure 11.4 Metaphyseal corner fracture involving anterior aspect of the distal femur. Images used with permission from VisualDx (www.visualdx.com)

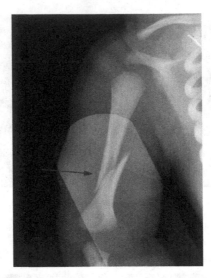

Figure 11.5 Displaced spiral fracture of the mid to distal humeral diaphysis. Images used with permission from VisualDx (www.visualdx.com)

Communicating With the Family

Clinicians should establish rapport with family members and caretakers, and establish that they are advocates for the patient, and suggest that all involved parties want what is best for the child. The family should also be informed that the police and/or CPS will be notified as clinicians are legally required to do so when suspicion of abuse exists.

Reporting

Of childhood injuries resulting in ED visits, 1.3%–15% are caused by abuse.[13] Physicians are mandated reporters of child abuse in all 50 states and are required by law to report all suspected cases of child abuse and neglect to the state. Mandatory reporting is required when there is "reasonable suspicion or reasonable cause to believe that abuse has occurred." Physicians have a broad and variable interpretation of what constitutes "reasonable suspicion," with some physicians even requiring 75% or more probability of abuse before they would report.[10] Nevertheless, reporting should occur as soon as child abuse is suspected.

The reporting process varies by state, but generally involves notification of the local CPS office or law enforcement agency of the child's name, and address of the child and family members; the child's age, sex, and primary language; the nature and extent of the child's injuries; the type of abuse or neglect; and prior history of abuse or neglect of the child or siblings. At the time of reporting (or sooner), it is useful to engage a multidisciplinary team when evaluating a child with suspected abuse, including social work, psychiatry, and the institution's child protection team (if one exists). After a report of suspected child maltreatment has been made, the child protection process is initiated and investigators will often come to the hospital to speak with the family and may go to the patient's home as well.

Substantiation means that there is sufficient evidence to believe that an act of abuse took place. CPS agencies investigate allegations of maltreatment; however, only 25% of all allegations are substantiated.[20]

Documentation

The documentation of child abuse important requires careful attention, as the clinical notes become medicolegal documents. Clear, objective, thorough, and precise language is important. Clinicians should not be judgmental, engage in conjecture, or draw conclusions that are not based upon facts. Documentation should include all details of the history, the parent–child interaction, physical exam findings, laboratory findings, consultant recommendations, and imaging reports, and the physical exam should include photos and/or detailed descriptions of any of the findings such as bruises and patterns of injury. All diagnostic study results must be included in the note along with a clinical impression and diagnostic reasoning.

Vignette Conclusion

This child had risk factors for maltreatment and a concerning physical exam. The clinician engaged the child protection team early who agreed with the plan to order imaging and blood work as well as consult ophthalmology to perform a retinal exam. His skeletal survey revealed multiple suspicious fractures for intentional injury and his head CT scan revealed a subdural hematoma that required observation in the intensive care unit. The clinician then spoke to the family about these concerns and reported the case to child protective services.

Pro-Tips

- Remember the red flags for child abuse and neglect.
- Cautiously employ risk factors with each patient to avoid bias.
- Take photographs of physical exam findings.
- When documenting your physical exam, do not make judgments or draw conclusions – be impartial and descriptive.
- Communicate well with the family as an advocate for your patient.
- Clinicians should be familiar with available child abuse resources and use them.
- Concerns should be reported to child protective services.

References

1. NYC Administration for Children's Services. What is child abuse/neglect? (cited April 29, 2022). Available from: www1 .nyc.gov/site/acs/child-welfare/what-is-child-abuse-neglect.page

2. Centers for Disease Control and Prevention. Fast Facts: Preventing Child Abuse & Neglect. 2022. Available from: www.cdc.gov /violenceprevention/childabuseandneglect/f astfact.html

3. The Child Abuse Prevention Center. Physical Neglect [California Penal Code Section 11165.2]. 2014 [cited April 27, 2022]. Available from: www .thecapcenter.org/why/types-of-abuse/phy sical-neglect

4. World Health Organization. Child maltreatment. 2020. Available from: www .who.int/news-room/fact-sheets/detail/child-maltreatment

5. Sedlak A, Mettenburg J, Basena M, Petta I, McPherson K, Greene A, Li S. *Fourth National Incidence Study of Child Abuse and Neglect (NIS-4) [Report to Congress]*. 2010. US Department of Health and Human Services, Administration for Children and Families. Available from: www.acf.hhs.gov/sites/default/files/documents/opre/nis4_report_congress_full_pdf_jan2010.pdf

6. Puls H, Bettenhausen J, Markham J, Walker J, Drake B, Kyler K, et al. Urban-rural residence and child physical abuse hospitalizations: a national incidence study. *J Pediatr*. 2019;205:230–235.

7. Boos S. Physical child abuse: recognition. 2022. UpToDate.

8. Centers for Disease Control and Prevention. Risk and Protective Factors. 2022. Available from: www.cdc.gov/violenceprevention/childabuseandneglect/riskprotectivefactors.html

9. McDonald KC. Child abuse: approach and management. Am Fam Physician. 2007;75(2):221–228

10. Boos S. Physical child abuse: diagnostic evaluation and management. 2021. UpToDate.

11. Henry K, Wood J. What's in a name? Sentinel injuries in abused infants. *Pediatr Radiol*. 2021;51,6:861–865.

12. Kodner C, Wetherton A. Diagnosis and management of physical abuse in children. *Am Fam Physician*. 2013;88(10):669–675.

13. Kellogg N, Committee on Child Abuse and Neglect. Evaluation of suspected child physical abuse. *Pediatrics*. 2007;119.

(6):1232–1241. Available from: https://publications.aap.org/pediatrics/article/119/6/1232/70638/Evaluation-of-Suspected-Child-Physical-Abuse

14. Shanahan M, Zolotor A, Parrish J, Barr R, Runyan D. National, regional, and state abusive head trauma: application of the CDC algorithm. *Pediatrics*. 2013;132(6): e1546–1553.

15. Christian C. Child abuse: evaluation and diagnosis of abusive head trauma in infants and children. 2021. UpToDate.

16. Lindberg D, Makoroff K, Harper N, Laskey A, Bechtel K, Deye K, Shapiro R, ULTRA Investigators. Utility of hepatic transaminases to recognize abuse in children. *Pediatrics*. 2009. 124(2):509–516. doi:10.1542/peds.2008-2348

17. Pierce M, Kaczor K, Aldridge S, O'Flynn J, Lorenz D. Bruising characteristics discriminating physical child abuse from accidental trauma. *Pediatrics*. 2010;125(4):861.

18. Adams JA, Harper K, Knudson S, Revilla J. Examination findings in legally confirmed child sexual abuse: it's normal to be normal. *Pediatrics*. 1994;94:310–317.

19. Boos S. Differential diagnosis of suspected child physical abuse. 2020. UpToDate.

20. Walsh W, Mattingly M. Understanding child abuse in rural and urban America: risk factors and maltreatment substantiation. 2012. Available from: https://scholars.unh.edu/cgi/viewcontent.cgi?article=1169&context=carsey

Further Reading

1. King W, Kiesel E, Simon H. Child abuse fatalities: are we missing opportunities for intervention? *Pediatr Emerg Care*. 2006;22(4):211–214. Available from: https://pubmed.ncbi.nlm.nih.gov/16651907/

2. The American College of Radiology. ACR-SPR Practice parameter for the perfroance and interpretation of skeletal surveys in children. 2021. Available from: www

.acr.org/-/media/ACR/Files/Practice-Parameters/Skeletal-Survey.pdf

3. Lawson M, Piel M, Simon M. Child maltreatment during the COVID-19 pandemic: consequences of parental job loss on psychological and physical abuse towards children. *Child Abuse Negl*. 2020;110(Pt 2):104709. doi:10.1016/j.chiabu.2020.104709

4. Griffith A. Parental burnout and child maltreatment during the COVID-19 pandemic. *J Fam Violence*. 2022;37(5):725–731. doi:10.1007/s10896-020-00172-2

5. Physical child abuse. 2022. VisualDx. Available from: www.visualdx.com/visualdx/diagnosis/physical+child+abuse?diagnosisId=51004&moduleId=102.

6. Bechtel K, Bennett B. Evaluation of sexual abuse in children and adolescents. 2021. UpToDate.

Care of Vulnerable Elders

Surriya Ahmad, Michael Stern, and Tony Rosen

Vignette

A 79-year-old woman is on a stretcher in the hallway. Per triage, she was dropped off at the emergency department (ED) by her grandson, but he is no longer at her bedside. She is unable to respond to questions in English, and it is unclear if she is altered or at her baseline. She appears cachectic, has on dirty clothes, and has bruising on both of her forearms. Her vital signs are within normal limits. She is not in distress. The reason she was brought to the ED is not clear.

- What is the approach to the evaluation and work-up for this patient?
- Are there important considerations?
- Are there resources that can be helpful In management in an urban ED?

Introduction

Most older adults in the US (as many as 80%) currently live in urban areas, with this fraction projected to increase.[1] In the US and other developed countries, these older adults living in cities are more likely to have poor overall self-reported health[2] and more commonly suffer from depression.[3] Racial minorities, who are more likely to live in urban areas, may be at particularly high risk for elder abuse. African Americans have been shown to have higher risk for financial exploitation and psychological abuse than other populations.[4,5] Homelessness is also increasingly common among older adults in urban settings.[6] The number of adults aged >65 experiencing homelessness is expected to triple between 2017 and 2030.[7]

As many as 10% of older adults living in the community (and more than 20% of nursing home residents) experience some form of abuse, neglect, or exploitation each year.[8] Elder mistreatment is under-recognized by emergency clinicians and under-reported to the authorities (Table 12.1). Elder mistreatment is thought to have a similar prevalence in urban and rural environments.[9–11] Despite this (and although not explored in detail), etiologies, risk factors, and opportunities for detection of elder mistreatment may differ in urban from other environments. Urban environments typically have smaller living spaces, and multiple family members, commonly several generations living together in close quarters. This living arrangement may increase the risk of elder mistreatment. In urban environments, neighbors live in closer proximity than in rural environments and may more commonly recognize mistreatment issues/activate 911. Homeless older adults are more likely to have mental illness and substance abuse issues, which increase elder mistreatment

Table 12.1 Types of Elder Mistreatment (Elder Abuse and Neglect)

Type	Definition	Examples
Physical abuse	Intentional use of physical force that may result in bodily injury, physical pain, or impairment	1. Slapping, hitting, kicking, pushing, pulling hair 2. Use of physical restraints, force-feeding 3. Burning, use of household objects as weapons, use of firearms and knives
Sexual abuse	Any type of sexual contact with an elderly person that is non-consensual or sexual contact with any person incapable of giving consent	1. Sexual assault or battery, such as rape, sodomy, coerced nudity, and sexually explicit photographing 2. Unwanted touching, verbal sexual advances 3. Indecent exposure
Neglect	Refusal or failure to fulfill any part of a person's obligations or duties to an elder, which may result in harm; may be intentional or unintentional	1. Withholding food, water, clothing, shelter, medications 2. Failure to ensure elder's personal hygiene or to provide physical aids, including walker, cane, glasses, hearing aids, dentures 3. Failure to ensure elder's personal safety and/or appropriate medical follow-up
Emotional/ psychological abuse	Intentional infliction of anguish, pain, or distress through verbal or non-verbal acts	1. Verbal berating, harassment, or intimidation 2. Threats of punishment or deprivation 3. Treating the older person like an infant 4. Isolating the older person from others
Abandonment	Desertion of an elderly person by an individual who has assumed responsibility for providing care for an elder or by a person with physical custody	
Financial/ material exploitation	Illegal or improper use of an older adult's money, property, or assets	1. Stealing money or belongings 2. Cashing an older adult's checks without permission and/or forging his or her signature 3. Coercing an older adult into signing contracts, changing a will, or assigning durable

Table 12.1 (cont.)

Type	Definition	Examples
		power of attorney against his or her wishes or when the older adult does not possess the mental capacity to do so
Self-neglect	Behavior of an older adult that threatens his/her own health or safety – excluding when an older adult who understands the consequences of his or her actions makes a conscious and voluntary decision to engage in acts that threaten his/her health or safety	1. Refusal or failure of an older adult to provide him- or herself with basic necessities, such as food, water, shelter, medications, and appropriate personal hygiene 2. Disregard for maintenance of safe home environment and/or hoarding

Adapted from National Center on Elder Abuse: Types of Abuse. Available at https://ncea.acl.gov/Suspect-Abuse/Abuse-Types.aspx

risk. Also, older adults who are living on the street or in shelters, given functional and cognitive limitations, may be particularly vulnerable to violence from others in their lives. Older adults living in rural environments are more likely to be isolated, which increases risk of mistreatment, and to have challenges with transportation to healthcare appointments and other interactions where abuse may be identified and reported.

Studies suggest that as few as 1 in 24 cases of elder abuse are reported to the authorities, and much of the associated adverse health outcomes and morbidity and mortality is likely due to this delay in identification and intervention.[8] Psychological/emotional and financial abuse and neglect are most commonly reported, while physical and sexual abuse are less commonly reported. Often, multiple types of elder mistreatment occur concurrently in the same patient.

Risk factors for becoming a victim or perpetrator of elder mistreatment are outlined in Table 12.2. It is important to keep in mind that many cases of elder mistreatment occur in the absence of risk factors and that overall, the phenomenon transgresses ethnic and socioeconomic boundaries such that no one is immune.

Assessment

Identifying Elder Abuse and Neglect in the Emergency Department

The ED visit provides an excellent opportunity to identify elder mistreatment, which may otherwise remain undiscovered. The nature of an ED encounter increases the potential for detection, as an older adult is typically assessed over several hours by multiple clinicians from different disciplines.[12] Despite the opportunity, emergency clinicians seldom identify and report elder abuse, supported by a study showing that elder abuse was diagnosed in only 0.013% of US ED visits.[13] Inadequate training, difficulty distinguishing between intentional and unintentional injuries, lack of time to conduct a thorough evaluation for mistreatment, concern about involvement in the legal system, a victim's unwillingness to report, and

Table 12.2 Risk Factors

Risk factors for becoming a victim

Functional dependence or disability
Poor physical health
Cognitive impairment/dementia
Poor mental health
Low income/socioeconomic status
Social isolation/low social support
Previous history of family violence
Previous traumatic event exposure
Substance abuse

Risk factors for becoming a perpetrator

Mental illness
Substance abuse
Caregiver stress
Previous history of family violence
Financial dependence on older adult

Data from references 12–16.

a victim's inability to report due to cognitive impairment are several reasons that exist for missed opportunity. One cannot identify what one is not thinking about, so increased awareness of elder mistreatment is the first step toward increased discovery in the ED setting.

When considering elder mistreatment, it is critical to assess an older adult without a family member/caregiver present. This may be particularly difficult in a crowded urban ED, a clinical setting where many patients are commonly examined on stretchers in the hallway. Older adults in urban environments more commonly speak a language other than English and have low English proficiency. This may isolate them and make it more challenging to seek help. This underscores the importance of using a professional rather than a family/informal translator and maintaining a high index of suspicion. When possible, obtain collateral information from others, including neighbors and doormen.

Clinical Features

Observation and Medical History

When beginning the evaluation, the ED clinician should observe patient/caregiver interactions if a caregiver is present at the bedside, watching for anything suggestive of potential mistreatment (see Table 12.3). Indicators of mistreatment in the medical history are shown in Table 12.4. Whenever possible, ED clinicians should attempt to separately interview the caregiver or suspected abuser and the patient, as this could potentially reveal discrepancies from the patient's history that may illuminate abuse or neglect. When conducting this interview, clinicians should avoid an accusatory or

Table 12.3 Observations from Older Adult/Caregiver Interactions That Should Raise Concern for Elder Mistreatment

- Older adult and caregiver provide conflicting accounts of events
- Caregiver interrupts/answers for the older adult
- Older adult seems fearful of or hostile toward caregiver
- Caregiver seems unengaged/inattentive in caring for the older adult
- Caregiver seems frustrated, tired, angry, or burdened by the older adult
- Caregiver seems overwhelmed by the older adult
- Caregiver seems to lack knowledge of the patient's care needs
- Evidence that the caregiver and/or older adult may be abusing alcohol or illicit drugs

Data from reference 12.

Table 12.4 Indicators from the Medical History of Possible Elder Mistreatment

- Unexplained injuries
- Past history of frequent injuries
- Elderly patient referred to as "accident prone"
- Delay between onset of medical illness or injury and seeking of medical attention
- Recurrent visits to the emergency department for similar injuries
- Using multiple physicians and emergency departments for care rather than one primary care physician ("doctor hopping or shopping")
- Non-compliance with medications, appointments, or physician directions

Data from reference 12.

critical approach, but rather frame it as a chance to find out more about the patient. When obtaining history, clinicians should assure the patient of privacy and confidentiality. Clinicians should explore in detail how any injuries occurred and consider asking directly about physical abuse if suspicion exists. In addition, clinicians should explore the patient's care needs, functional status, cognition, and safety of the home environment, and may ask whether the patient feels socially isolated. During history taking, ED clinicians should observe for signs in the patient's behavior that suggest the potential for abuse and neglect, including fear, anxiety, low self-esteem, and poor eye contact. Attempting to speak to the patient is particularly important, even if it appears as though they will not be able to provide a history, as subtle clues may be identified. A recent study found that a vast majority of patients with mild cognitive impairment were able to accurately report elder abuse.[14] In fact, cognitive impairment/dementia is an independent risk factor for elder mistreatment. If an older adult is unable to provide a history, emergency clinicians should seek collateral history from the primary care clinician, family members, neighbors, visiting nurses, or home health aides as appropriate.

Physical Exam

Performing a comprehensive physical exam in conjunction with the interview is essential to adequately evaluate for elder mistreatment (see Table 12.5). Emergency department clinicians concerned about mistreatment should document their findings in detail, including complete descriptions of all physical findings including even minor injuries, and should consider photographing findings or using a body diagram/traumagram.

Laboratory Testing and Imaging

No one blood or urine test is definitively diagnostic for elder mistreatment, although certain findings may raise or increase suspicion, including anemia, dehydration, malnutrition, hypothermia/hyperthermia, and rhabdomyolysis.[15] Emergency department clinicians should consider checking prescription medication and illicit drug levels, as low or undetectable levels may indicate withholding by a caregiver. Additionally, elevated drug levels may indicate overdose, while the presence of toxins of drugs that have not been prescribed may indicate poisoning.[15]

Table 12.5 Physical Signs Suspicious for Potential Elder Abuse or Neglect

Physical abuse

Bruising in atypical locations (not over bony prominences/on lateral arms, back, face, ears, or neck)

Patterned injuries (bite marks or injury consistent with the shape of a belt buckle, fingertip, or other object)

Wrist or ankle lesions or scars (suggesting inappropriate restraints)

Burns (particularly stocking/glove pattern suggesting forced immersion or cigarette pattern)

Multiple fractures or bruises of different ages

Traumatic alopecia or scalp hematomas

Subconjunctival, vitreous, or retinal ophthalmic hemorrhages

Intraoral soft tissue injuries

Sexual abuse

Genital, rectal, or oral trauma (including erythema, bruising, lacerations)

Evidence of sexually transmitted disease

Neglect

Cachexia/malnutrition

Dehydration

Pressure sores/decubitus ulcers

Poor body hygiene, unchanged diaper

Dirty, severely worn clothing

Elongated toenails

Poor oral hygiene

Data from references 12, 19–23, 25, 26.

Limited radiology literature exists describing potential imaging correlates of elder mistreatment.[16-18] Findings suggestive of mistreatment may include co-occurring old and new fractures, high injury fractures with low energy mechanism, distal ulnar diaphyseal fractures, and small bowel hematomas.[16-18] The ED clinician should communicate any suspicion for elder mistreatment to the radiologist and ask them to focus on whether the imaging findings are consistent with the purported history. Clinicians may also consider additional screening imaging tests, including maxillofacial computed tomography (CT) scan and chest x-ray, to evaluate for acute and chronic fractures.

Screening

Screening for elder mistreatment is a standardized assessment whose goal is to increase identification in a historically under-detected population. Most common screening consists of a single question about home safety, and it is generally accepted that this single question is inadequate and often represents a missed opportunity for identification.[19] Screening may be universal or targeted. The ED Senior Abuse Identification tool (ED Senior AID) has been validated for use in the ED.[20-22] The Emergency Medicine Screening and Response Tool (EM-SART) is a promising tool that includes a brief initial 2–3 question screen and administration of the full ED Senior AID Tool if positive).[19,20] This addresses the issue that completing the ED Senior AID tool on all patients would be very time-consuming. Space issues in many crowded urban EDs may make screening in a private setting without a family member/caregiver present challenging or even impossible. Language and cultural issues for patients may make screening with questions more challenging.

Universal screening might be ideal to increase identification, but it may not be practical in understaffed, busy urban EDs – in this case, ED clinicians need to consider the potential that abuse is occurring contributing to an older adult's presentation and explore more deeply when appropriate.

Management

The first step of treatment is addressing acute traumatic, medical, and psychological issues. If an elder mistreatment victim is in immediate danger, the patient should be prevented from having any contact with the suspected abuser, which may require a security watch for the patient and having the abuser removed from the ED. Alerting law enforcement, hospital social workers, and administrators should be considered. Alternate living arrangements may need to be arranged for the patient to ensure safety, and, if no reliable options are available, the patient may require hospital admission.

If the patient refuses intervention, the emergency clinician must determine whether the patient has the capacity to make this decision, and a psychiatric consultation may be helpful in these particular cases. If an older adult is deemed to have capacity, their wishes must be honored, including returning to an abusive situation. The ED clinician should educate the patient about the potential for escalation in violence and abuse and provide appropriate referral information for future use. If an older adult does not have decision-making capacity, an ED clinician should proceed with treatments that are in the patient's best interest, including hospitalization if appropriate. In cases where a patient does not have decision-making capacity, and the suspected abuser is the patient's official health care proxy or power of attorney, the ED clinician should involve hospital administration, legal, and ethics to assist with healthcare decision-making and consideration of pursing legal guardianship.

If the patient wants to return home and may be safely discharged, the ED clinician should coordinate with the patient's primary care clinician to ensure an appropriate longitudinal follow-up plan.

Urban EDs are more likely than rural EDs to have social workers/care coordinators, and involving these professionals, who have expertise in socio-medical issues and are most familiar with available services/resources in the care of these vulnerable older adults, is critical. Notably, for the many EDs where these professionals are only available during business hours, it is usually worth holding the older adult in the ED overnight until the morning for assessment than rather than discharging during the night.

Urban environments likely have a broader range of services available to vulnerable older adults than rural environments, and ED clinicians should keep these in mind when considering how to make disposition as safe as possible. These may include, in addition to Adult Protective Services (APS), community-based agencies, respite and caregiver support programs, senior centers, meals on wheels, and friendly visitors. Most ED clinicians are likely not aware of these services or how to connect older adults to them. Free online tools, such as the website www.findhelp.org, developed by AuntBertha.com, can be used to find available social services by zip code. In urban EDs where social workers or care coordinators are not available during nights and weekends or after hours, this may be particularly helpful.

As many urban older adults have low English proficiency, it is important to keep in mind that providing effective assistance depends on ensuring that an older adult can receive services in a language they understand. In urban environments, particularly in safety net public hospital EDs, older adults are less likely than in rural communities to be well-connected to a primary care clinician. This is a challenge and makes patient navigator and other post-discharge follow-up programs critical to optimize safety.

Trauma-Informed Care

Providing trauma-informed care focuses on the patient's need for safety, respect, and acceptance. ED clinicians should try to maximize victim agency and control while minimizing re-traumatization through treatment. Recommended bedside strategies[23] include:

- Using language that is easily interpreted neutral, and unintimidating
- Limiting the number of times a victim is asked to talk about the assault
- Avoiding words such as violence, abuse, or criminal behavior if the victim does not initially conceive of what has occurred as abusive or criminal
- Asking permission before touching a potential victim
- Maintaining the victim's privacy and confidentiality
- Offering the support of an advocate if available
- Being mindful of culturally specific expectations regarding interactions between older adult patients and younger care clinicians

Documentation

Thorough and accurate documentation of the history and physical examination findings can help ensure that there is justice for victims in cases that result in legal action. The ED clinician should document the history in the patient's own words if possible. Pertinent social history, such as the patient's functional status, the caregiver's relationship to the patient, and living arrangements, should be included. General appearance on initial arrival to the ED should be described, including injuries of any type. Clinicians should consider using a body diagram/traumagram when possible to enhance precision of physical finding documentation (see physical exam section above).[24] Attempts should be made to include photographs of all injuries in the medical record. By standardizing the documentation used in the ED as much as possible, researchers may have greater success identifying injury patterns from chart reviews.

Reporting

ED clinicians should report even potential cases of elder mistreatment to the appropriate authorities, as suspicion is all that is needed to report. Reports for community-dwelling older adults are made to APS in most US urban communities

It is important to note that, in most US states, APS may only investigate cases where an older adult has either cognitive or functional impairment. Emergency department clinicians should be aware that APS functions differently than Child Protective Services.[8] In most cases, APS will not open their investigation while a patient is in the ED or an in-patient unit in the hospital, both of which are considered safe environments. Rather, they will wait until after the patient's discharge from the hospital. If an ED clinician is concerned about a patient's immediate safety or that a crime has been committed, involving local law enforcement should be considered.[8] Clinicians should check for policies in their state and county.

For any suspicion or identification of elder mistreatment in nursing home patients, ED clinicians should report to the long-term care ombudsman in their state, the state's Department of Health, or APS for further investigation.

Team-Based Multidisciplinary Approach

A team based multidisciplinary approach[25] in the ED can be fundamental in optimizing chances for detection of elder mistreatment in the ED, and for management of next steps post detection. Components include emergency medical services (EMS), the triage team, nursing interactions at bedside, techs, radiologists, clerks, transport, and social work to aid in providing counseling, safety planning, and resources to patient and caregiver.

Multidisciplinary response teams may be helpful in ensuring safety and justice for vulnerable older adults. While launching and sustaining these teams requires resources, urban receiving hospitals, many of which have already active, strong programs for victims of child abuse and intimate partner violence, may be the optimal environments in a community in which to build them. State and federal funders of these other programs for different populations have also supported ED-based elder abuse response teams. Outcomes of ED-based elder mistreatment consultation response teams[26] on enhancing detection of elder mistreatment, similar to those used for cases of child abuse, are being studied.

COVID 19

During the COVID 19 pandemic, a previously undescribed type of elder abuse occurred. A vulnerable older adult, often with multiple medical problems that increased their risk of a poor outcome if they contracted COVID 19, lived with and could not avoid close contact with a younger family member who, despite the older adult's requests, refused to take precautions to avoid COVID 19 exposure that might lead to transmission to the vulnerable older adult. These behaviors caused substantial psychological stress for many older adults and led to arguments and escalation in many cases. This was likely more common in urban settings, with smaller living spaces making avoiding cohabitants much more difficult. The ability to adequately protect against infectious exposure is an important component of home safety during this and any future pandemic.

Self-Neglect

Self-neglect is the most common form of elder mistreatment reported to social services. It does not involve another person as the perpetrator. It includes behaviors in which an older adult threatens his/her own health or safety by failing to perform or refusing assistance with essential self-care, including eating (resulting in malnutrition), failure to take necessary medications, inattention to personal hygiene, hoarding, and not maintaining a safe home environment. Comorbid conditions including cognitive dysfunction, psychiatric illness, and substance abuse disorders are often present. Self-neglect is associated with increased mortality. Recognition of self-neglect by ED clinicians is critical, as it may be the only opportunity outside the home for a healthcare professional to recognize this dangerous syndrome. Often, admission to the hospital is required to ensure an ultimate safe disposition.[8]

One challenge for clinicians when considering how to optimally manage potential self-neglect in an urban setting is keeping in mind that, in the communal apartment living that is common in urban environments, an unsafe home environment with fire hazards, vermin infestation, or mold poses a threat not only to the older adult but also to their neighbors in other apartments in the same building. This should be taken into account when deciding next steps including reporting.

Vignette Conclusion

The patient speaks Polish, is hard of hearing, and has mild cognitive impairment based on electronic health record information from another hospital. Using a video translator and headphones, the team obtains history that her grandson, who has been her primary caregiver, has relapsed on alcohol and other drugs. By calling one of the patient's daughters, who lives in another state, and her primary care physician, the team learns that they are both very concerned about her health and safety. They do not think her grandson is giving her regular medications, which include phenytoin. Her phenytoin level is low, supporting this. She also has been prescribed hydrocodone for chronic back pain, and there is concern that her grandson is diverting it for his own use. The patient's sodium level is elevated, suggesting dehydration, and her albumin is very low, suggesting potential malnutrition. The patient has a decubitus ulcer with significant surrounding maceration. The patient is unable to explain the bruises on her forearms. Chest x-ray finds multiple old rib fractures in various stages of healing. This raises concern for potential physical abuse. The ED social worker is deeply involved in the care of this patient and in decision-making about next steps. The patient is admitted to the hospital with a plan to develop a safe discharge plan, including home health care, moving in with another family member, and a referral to Adult Protective Services.

Pro-Tips

- Elder abuse is common and has serious health consequences – ED clinicians should consider this when assessing urban-dwelling older adults.
- It is critical to assess an older adult without a family member/caregiver present and that a professional translator is used with hearing assistance as needed.
- Signs suggestive of potential elder abuse and neglect exist in physical examination, and older adults should be examined head to toe.
- Obtaining collateral from family, caregivers, neighbors, outpatient clinicians, and others may provide important information about a patient.
- Emergency department management of elder abuse should include: complete documentation, treating acute issues, ensuring patient safety (which may involve admission to the hospital for safety), and proper reporting to the authorities.
- Social workers and care coordinators have expertise in socio-medical issues and are most familiar with available services/resources in the care of these vulnerable older adults – involve them early.

References

1. Beard JR, Petitot C. Ageing and urbanization: can cities be designed to foster active ageing? *Public Health Rev.* 2010;32 (2):427–450. doi: 10.1007/BF03391610.

2. Cohen SA, Cook SK, Sando TA, Sabik NJ. What aspects of rural life contribute to rural–urban health disparities in older adults? Evidence from a national survey. *J Rural Health.* 2018;34(3):293–303.

3. Purtle J, Nelson KL, Yang Y, Langellier B, Stankov I, Diez Roux AV. Urban–rural differences in older adult depression: a systematic review and meta-analysis of comparative studies. *Am J Prev Med.* 2019;56(4):603–613. doi: https://doi.org/10 .1016/j.amepre.2018.11.008.

4. Pillemer K, Burnes D, Riffin C, Lachs MS. Elder abuse: global situation, risk factors, and prevention strategies. *Gerontologist* 2016;56(Suppl 2):S194–205. doi: 10.1093/ geront/gnw004.

5. Dong XQ. Elder abuse: systematic review and implications for practice. *J Am Geriatr Soc.* 2015;63(6):1214–1238. doi: 10.1111/ jgs.13454.

6. Stergiopoulos V, Herrmann N. Old and homeless: a review and survey of older adults who use shelters in an urban setting. *Can J Psychiatry.* 2003;48(6):374–380. doi: 10.1177/070674370304800603.

7. Ureste P, Smith W, Morgan S. Caring for older adults experiencing homelessness in the inpatient psychiatry setting: challenges and recommendations. *Am J Geriatr Psychiatry.* 2022;30(4, Suppl):S12–S13. doi: https://doi.org/10.1016/j.jagp.2022.01.270.

8. Rosen, T. Chapter 181: Geriatric abuse and neglect. In Walls R, Hockberger R, Gausche-Hill M, Erickson TB, Wilcox SR (eds.). *Rosen's Emergency Medicine: Concepts and Clinical Practice*, 10th ed. Elsevier, 2022.

9. Warren A, Blundell B. Addressing elder abuse in rural and remote communities: social policy, prevention and responses. *J Elder Abuse Neglect*. 2019;31(4–5):424–436. doi: 10.1080/08946566.2019.1663333.

10. Acierno R, Hernandez MA, Amstadter AB, Resnick HS, Steve K, Muzzy W, Kilpatrick DG. Prevalence and correlates of emotional, physical, sexual, and financial abuse and potential neglect in the United States: the National Elder mistreatment Study. *Am J Public Health*. 2010;100(2):292–277. doi: 10.2105/AJPH.2009.163089.

11. Amstadter AB, Zajac K, Strachan M, Hernandez MA, Kilpatrick DG, Acierno R. Prevalence and correlates of elder mistreatment in South Carolina: the South Carolina Elder Mistreatment Study. *J Interpers Violence*. 2011;26(15):2947–2972. doi: 10.1177/0886260510390959.

12. Rosen T, Stern ME, Elman A, Mulcare MR. Identifying and initiating intervention for elder abuse and neglect in the emergency department. *Clin Geriatr Med*. 2018;34:435–451.

13. Evans CS, Hunold KM, Rosen T, Platts-Mills TF. Diagnosis of elder abuse in U.S. emergency departments. *J Am Geriatr Soc*. 2017;65:91–97.

14. Richmond NL, Zimmerman S, Reeve, BB, Dayaa JA, Davis ME, Bowen SB, Iasiello JA, Stemerman R, Shams RB, Haukoos JS, Sloane PD, Travers D, Mosqueda LA, McLean SA, Platts-Mills TF. Ability of older adults to report elder abuse: an emergency department–based cross-sectional study. *J Am Geriatr Soc*. 2020;68:170–175.

15. LoFaso VM, Rosen T. Medical and laboratory indicators of elder abuse and neglect. *Clin Geriatr Med*. 2014;30:713–728.

16. Murphy K, Waa S, Jaffer H, Sauter A, Chan A. A literature review of findings in physical elder abuse. *Can Assoc Radiol J*. 2013;64:10–14.

17. Rosen T, Bloemen EM, Harpe J, Sanchez AM, Mennitt KW, McCarthy TJ, Nicola R, Murphy K, LoFaso VM, Flomenbaum N, Lachs MS. Radiologists' training, experience, and attitudes about elder abuse detection. *AJR Am J Roentgenol*. 2016;207:1210–1214.

18. Wong NZ, Rosen T, Sanchez AM, Bloemen EM, Mennitt KW, Hentel K, Nicola R, Murphy K, LoFaso VM, Flomenbaum N, Lachs MS. Imaging findings in elder abuse: a role for radiologists in detection. *Can Assoc Radiol J*. 2017;68:16–20.

19. Rosen T, Platts-Mills TF, Fulmer T. Screening for elder mistreatment in emergency departments: current progress and recommendations for next steps. *J Elder Abuse Negl*. 2020;32(3):295–315.

20. Platts-Mills TF, Sivers-Teixeira T, Encarnacion A, Tanksley B, Olsen B. EM-SART: a scalable elder mistreatment screening and response tool for emergency departments. *Generations: J Am Soc Aging*. 2020;44(1):51–58.

21. Platts-Mills TF, Hurka-Richardson K, Shams RB, et al. Multicenter validation of an emergency department-based screening tool to identify elder abuse. *Ann Emerg Med*. 2020;76(3):280–290. doi: 10.1016/j.annemergmed.2020.07.005.

22. Platts-Mills TF, Dayaa JA, Reeve BB, Krajick K, Mosqueda L, Haukoos JS, Patel MD, Mulford CF, McLean SA, Sloane PD, Travers D, Zimmerman S. Development of the emergency department senior abuse identification (ED Senior AID) tool. *J Elder Abuse Negl*. 2018;30:247–270.

23. Ramsey-Klawsnik H, Miller E. Polyvictimization in later life: trauma-informed best practices. *J Elder Abuse Negl*. 2017;29:339–350.

24. Kogan AC, Rosen T, Navarro A, Homeier D, Chennapan K, Mosqueda L. Developing the Geriatric Injury Documentation Tool (Geri-IDT) to improve documentation of physical findings in injured older adults. *J Gen Intern Med*. 2019;34(4):567–574.

25. Rosen T, Hargarten S, Flomenbaum NE, Platts-Mills TF. Identifying elder abuse in the emergency department: toward a multidisciplinary team-based approach. *Ann Emerg Med.* 2016;68:378–382.

26. Rosen T, Mehta-Naik N, Elman A, Mulcare MR, Stern ME, Clark S, Sharma R, LoFaso VM, Breckman R, Lachs M, Needell N. Improving quality of care in hospitals for victims of elder mistreatment: development of the vulnerable elder protection team. *Jt Comm J Qual Patient Saf.* 2018;44:164–171.

Chapter 13

Civil Unrest: Caring for Police and Protesters

Scott A. Goldberg and Stephen G. DeVries

Vignette 1

Last night, after the shooting of an unarmed civilian by police, several spontaneous protests broke out in a mid-sized Midwestern city. A community hospital downtown treated multiple patients with minor injuries – a police officer with heat stroke, two protestors with blunt trauma from rubber bullets, and three protestors experiencing vision changes, burning eyes, and wheezing after exposure to a tear gas grenade.

Local law enforcement warns all hospitals in the city to prepare for larger protests in the coming days.

- What are the key hospital preparedness priorities?
- What specific steps should be taken to mobilize resources?

Vignette 2

At 11:30 p.m. that same evening, the local news channel announces that crowds are growing downtown, and 15 minutes later, reports of a physical confrontation between police and protestors are received by the closest receiving emergency department (ED). Over the next few hours, several patients arrive. Three patients are in acute respiratory distress after exposure to a crowd dispersal agent, and four protestors (now under arrest) require medical clearance after altercations with law enforcement. A patient with a Taser barb embedded in the left side of the chest is coming in. A police officer was exposed to an unknown substance believed to be urine and will arrive in her own vehicle. In addition, dozens of patients have walked into the hospital and are checking in with severe eye pain and coughing. A few have reported that they were exposed to a "smoke grenade" that was thrown into a building.

- Given that the number of patients is increasing and their injuries are more severe than anticipated, what additional steps can be taken to support resource mobilization and hospital response?
- How should arriving patients be triaged and prioritized?
- What are the key concerns when managing patients with potential contamination from crowd dispersal agents?

Introduction

Civil unrest, or civil disorder, is defined in United States statute as "any public disturbance involving acts of violence by assemblage of three or more persons, which causes an immediate danger of or results in damage or injury to the property or person of any other individual."[1] Such events may involve protests or demonstrations in response to political or economic activities, responses to concerts or sporting events, or in response to controversial actions by law enforcement.

While still uncommon, incidents of civil unrest are increasing in frequency across the United States. During episodes of civil unrest, injuries may occur either in isolation or in associated interactions with law enforcement personnel. Unfortunately, data on the incidence of injury or ED presentation associated with episodes of civil unrest are limited.[2,3] Nevertheless, it is important for the urban emergency medicine practitioner to be familiar with the basic principles of medical care during episodes of civil unrest, as well as to have a fundamental understanding of the management of common injuries associated with law enforcement interactions.

Most patients will have patterns of injury that the ED clinician can readily diagnose and manage. However, there are some specific patterns of injury that are unique to protests and encounters with law enforcement that warrant further examination. We will highlight several of these here, including general principles of ED readiness and field response.

General Principles of Emergency Department Care

Planning and preparation are essential components of the ED response during periods of civil unrest. Often, the department will have advanced warning of potential demonstrations or protests or have awareness of other mass gatherings with the potential for violence. However, advanced notification may be limited, as is the case with spontaneous riots occurring after a sporting event. Lessons learned from recent events highlight the importance of an institutional emergency response plan. In anticipation of common injuries associated with civil unrest, efforts should be made to secure additional trauma resources and intensive care unit space. Decontamination supplies should be readied, and institutions may choose to mobilize their decontamination equipment and teams.[4] In an effort to protect patients and staff, facility lockdown procedures should be considered in collaboration with security and law enforcement personnel.[5]

While specific patterns of injury are described in more detail below, care in the ED generally follows usual principles of emergency medical care. Whenever possible, patients with differing political viewpoints should be placed in different areas of the department to minimize potential for conflict. Further, law enforcement may be present in the ED as either patients or in an investigatory capacity. This law enforcement presence may be contentious and negatively impact care.[6] Efforts should be made to limit interactions between law enforcement personnel and other patients unless required for medical care or prevailing regulatory requirements. Law enforcement and media may also present to the ED inquiring about specific patients. ED physicians should not disclose information to law enforcement except that which is permitted by institutional policy or required by law.[7] Information should never be shared with the media. All media inquiries should be referred to the institution's public information officer (PIO). Identifying the PIO ahead of time, and having a defined media communication strategy, is helpful.

A careful belongings search should be conducted on all patients entering the ED, while maintaining patient autonomy and respecting dignity. Emergency department documentation may be referenced in later legal actions involving both law enforcement and protesters. While ED documentation should always follow best practices for medical documentation, in cases involving civil unrest it is especially important that clinical documentation should be factual and remain unbiased, as these records may be used in future legal proceedings.[8] Judgment statements against either law enforcement or protestors should be avoided, and documentation must remain neutral. A careful and thorough description of any symptoms and physical exam findings is essential.

Patterns of Illness and Injury

Typical Patterns of Injury

Blunt trauma is the major injury pattern during civil unrest, although occasionally firearm injuries do occur. Most injuries will be typical traumatic injuries from physical altercations, falls, or other minor traumatic mechanisms, and these injuries should be treated in line with usual emergency medicine practice. Use of force by law enforcement personnel typically results in minor trauma from unarmed physical force,[9,10] although some traumatic mechanisms are unique to civil unrest. Reports from recent demonstrations and protests have highlighted the use of projectiles including frozen water bottles, canned goods, bricks, and other objects intended to inflict blunt traumatic injury. The burden of injury will vary depending on personal protective equipment (PPE) worn by law enforcement personnel.

There have been recent reports of demonstrators using body fluids including urine and feces as projectiles directed at law enforcement. While these events are emotionally disturbing, the risk of contracting communicable diseases is negligible provided that the officer is wearing PPE including a basic dress uniform and eye protection. Any exposed skin should be copiously irrigated. A discussion on the risks and benefits of post-exposure prophylaxis can be made on a case-by-case basis, although will not be indicated in most cases.

Use of canines in support of law enforcement personnel is uncommon in civil unrest but does occur. When injury occurs as a result of the use of law enforcement canines, these injuries have the potential to be severe.[9] Significant injury should be treated as penetrating trauma and managed accordingly. Emergency department treatment for less-significant injury should include copious wound irrigation and management consistent with usual care for canine bite injuries, including antibiotics for higher-risk patients or wounds or for wounds undergoing primary closure. The vaccination status of law enforcement canines should be known and can be confirmed by the involved law enforcement personnel. An additional consideration associated with canine use of force is psychological and emotional. An after-action report from Ferguson, MO cited the use of canines as an ineffective crowd control strategy that evoked strong negative emotions in observing citizens and protestors.[11]

Public safety personnel may be providing support for extended periods of time, often exposed to inclement weather conditions. Environmental factors may be compounded by heavy PPE including body armor. Depending on patient-specific factors including age, fitness level, comorbid medical conditions, and event duration, officers may suffer heat- or cold-related illness. Public safety personnel should be encouraged to hydrate and take frequent rests during work details, especially in extreme weather conditions. While most symptoms will be self-limiting and can be treated on scene, occasionally law enforcement personnel may require medical evaluation and may present to the ED with symptoms of heat stress including fatigue and dehydration. Treatment is largely symptomatic, including cooling, hydration, and supportive care.

Also unique to ED presentations during times of civil unrest are injuries and illness resulting from less-lethal use of law enforcement force. Some entities, including the US Department of Defense and the North Atlantic Treaty Organization, still refer to these weapons as "non-lethal," although the broader literature generally uses the United Nations-preferred term "less-lethal" on the premise that any weapon has the potential to cause death or serious injury. Injuries from less-lethal weapons are common reasons for ED presentation after civil unrest. These weapons include blunt force projectiles, chemical crowd dispersal agents, and sound, laser, and electrical devices. To ensure proper management, emergency clinicians must understand not only the typical injury patterns and complications caused by these weapons, but also the basic characteristics of the weapons themselves. Below, we discuss the three categories of less-lethal weapons most often deployed during civil unrest: projectiles, crowd dispersal agents, and electrical devices.

Kinetic Impact Projectiles

Traditional firearms are designed to inflict trauma through penetrating injury. Conversely, kinetic impact projectiles, or KIPs, are blunt-force projectiles designed to inflict pain and irritation through the transfer of kinetic energy and resultant blunt injury. Projectiles may be made of wood, rubber, or plastic and are designed to deter without inflicting permanent injury. However, while these projectiles are not intended to penetrate, penetrating injuries do occur, particularly on impact to the head, face, and neck, and are a cause of significant morbidity and mortality.[12]

Kinetic impact projectiles come in many varieties. Bean bags are relatively soft, but projectiles may also be made of metal with a rubber coating, pure rubber, wood, or plastic. Importantly, these weapons are designed for use at a narrow range of distances. The energy of these projectiles quickly dissipates over distance; shot from too far away, they may have little to no effect. Shot too close, they could cause serious injury or death. These devices are less accurate than ordinary bullets, increasing potential for unintended injuries.

Recent studies of injury patterns from less-lethal weapons have focused on the civil unrest in Hong Kong in 2019 and 2020 (the Anti-Extradition Law Amendment Bill Movement), in France in 2018 and 2019 (the Yellow Vest protests), and in the United States after the murder of George Floyd in May 2020. Systematic studies of injury patterns due to KIPs are limited, but existing data suggest that these weapons are not as safe as once thought.[13] One large-scale review of injuries, deaths, and permanent disabilities caused by projectiles included injury data for 1984 people between 1990 and 2017. Across six geopolitical regions worldwide, there were 53 fatalities and 15% of survivors suffered severe disability.[12]

Up to 82% of permanently disabling injuries result from strikes to the head or face.[12] As such, emergency clinicians should perform careful assessment for ocular injuries and have a low threshold for computed tomography (CT) of the face. A recent series from France described numerous severe facial injuries caused by rubber bullets, including orbital blowout fractures.[14] Immediate interventions including lateral canthotomy and cantholysis may be indicated to preserve eyesight in the case of compromised vision and retrobulbar injury. Early involvement of an ophthalmologist in the case of vision compromise from KIPs is recommended.

As with other injuries, emergency clinicians must tailor the diagnostic strategy to the observed trauma burden. In rare cases, though, what appears to be a relatively minor injury from a blunt-force projectile can cause death. In a tragic case report, a man was struck by a rubber projectile shot from a distance of 7 m away and immediately collapsed with an initial rhythm of asystole.[15] The cause of death was determined to be commotio cordis, a condition in which blunt trauma to the chest wall results in a potentially fatal arrhythmia.[16] Emergency clinicians should be cognizant of the worst-case scenario, whether it be commotio cordis, lung contusion, or another serious complication.

Conducted Electrical Weapons

Also known as electroshock weapons, this class of weapons sends an electrical arc between electrodes to cause involuntary muscle contraction and intense pain in a subject. There are many types and brands of conducted electrical weapon (CEW) on the market, but the two that emergency clinicians in the United States will encounter most frequently are the stun gun and Taser (Thomas A. Swift Electronic Rifle). With a stun gun, the user must physically place the weapon against the subject to discharge it. From a law enforcement perspective, the obvious disadvantage of this weapon is that it puts the officer in potential danger by requiring them to be in extremely close physical proximity to the subject. Perhaps for this reason, the more common CEW used by law enforcement in the United States is the Taser. A Taser enables law enforcement to fire barbed electrodes at subjects up to 25 feet away. Unlike a stun gun, some distance must be present for the Taser barbs to appropriately deploy allowing for conduction of the intended electric arc.

Electroshock weapons discharge bursts of high-frequency, low-amperage current that by design ensures that the electrical energy stays at the surface of the body and does not penetrate into deeper organs.[17,18] They are generally considered to be quite safe, although evaluating their safety in a robust quantitative manner is complicated by the fact that there is no mandatory or centralized reporting procedure for Taser use and outcomes in the United States. For emergency clinicians treating patients injured by stun gun discharges, the main considerations are injuries from fall, and – though much less likely – injuries secondary to the electricity. In evaluating a Taser victim, the emergency clinician must also consider damage from the penetrating barb, as well as possible foreign body removal.

Studies of Taser-related morbidity and mortality suggest that mortality, when it does occur, is generally associated to comorbid medical conditions such as underlying arrhythmia, or unrelated factors such as intoxication.[19] Recent studies of thousands of police use-of-force events have affirmed that when law enforcement use Tasers in place of physical force, risk of injury decreases for both police and suspects.[20] With regard to cardiac risk specifically, even when probes are lodged in locations that could produce a trans-cardiac discharge vector, Taser use does not seem to cause cardiac dysrhythmia, although this is a subject of ongoing study.[21] In an awake, alert patient with a CEW exposure of up to 15 s, the available literature does not support performance of any laboratory studies, electrocardiography, or prolonged observation.[22]

When a Taser is fired at a subject, two electrodes on wires with barbs of approximately 4 mm length attach to the subject's clothes or skin.[17] Law enforcement officers are often trained to remove Taser barbs, so emergency clinicians will rarely see patients presenting for embedded barb removal unless there are comorbid traumatic injuries. However, if required, barb removal is simple: tug sharply on the barb, after stretching the surrounding skin taut. If this technique is not successful, a small incision can be made over the barb to make it easier to remove. Law enforcement will usually cut wires from the Taser before presentation, but if not, clinicians should cut these before barb removal. There are no absolute contraindications to barb removal, although a specialist should be consulted for barbs lodged in the eye or genitals, especially if there is concern that removal could cause greater trauma to the area.

Crowd Dispersal Agents

Law enforcement will sometimes use chemical agents to control or break up crowds or subdue individuals. Also known as lacrimators, riot control agents, harassing agents, tear gas, or incapacitating agents, they are generally safe, but in rare cases they may cause serious complications (Table 13.1). The three agents most frequently used by law enforcement in the United States are oleoresin capsicum (OC, also known as pepper spray), 2-chloroacetophenone (CN, also known as Mace), and o-chlorobenzylidene malonitrile (CS).[23] Today, law enforcement in the United States use mostly CS and OC. The purpose of these agents is to temporarily incapacitate a subject or group of subjects without causing permanent harm. Upon exposure to the mucous membranes of the human eye, nose, respiratory tract, and mouth, as well as to a lesser extent the skin, the most common effect of these three crowd dispersal agents is irritation. Subjects exposed to these agents also experience severe pain, difficulty seeing due to lacrimation and blepharospasm, disorientation, and sensation of respiratory distress.[24] The effects are immediate, but most patients – even those who initially present in severe discomfort – recover quickly after removal and decontamination from the offending agent. Symptoms associated with exposure to most crowd dispersal agents dissipate quickly on evacuation of the area, and as such are effective in motivating individuals to clear an area in which they may be congregating.

Crowd dispersal agents can be deployed through a variety of mechanisms. While often referred to as "tear gas," these agents are actually fine particulates that are aerosolized in smoke or spray at the time of dispersal. Pepper spray generally refers to a hand-held OC system that is designed to incapacitate one or several subjects, rather than a large crowd. In these cases, the active agent is never actually aerosolized, but instead discharged as a liquid directly at the target. Air-powered guns can also deploy small pellets filled with OC that release the substance when striking a target. By contrast, aerosolized CS may affect a much

Table 13.1 Typical Symptoms and Management of Exposure to Crowd Dispersal Agents

Symptom	Management
Mild respiratory distress even after decontamination	Humidified oxygen
Excessive secretions	Suctioning
Severe respiratory distress (usually from laryngospasm)	Intubation
Stridor or other sings of upper airway compromise	Inhaled racemic epinephrine Bronchoscopy for the critical patient
Pulmonary edema	Supplemental oxygen, advise rest from physical activity when stable for discharge
Lower airway symptoms (wheezing)	Similar to asthma exacerbation (short-acting beta-2 agonist and systemic steroids)

larger area and many more people, potentially leading to a much higher volume of patients in nearby EDs. CS is generally deployed through grenades or other projectile cartridges, which aerosolize the irritant substance on detonation. While the irritant itself is the intended deterrent, the cartridge or pellet can also cause injury through blunt trauma. Although generally safe, exposure to high concentrations or for long periods of time can be associated with morbidity or mortality. In nearly all case reports of significant injury and death from exposure to crowd dispersal agents, there are two commonalities: exposure in a confined area and/or exposure for a long period of time.

Of the three crowd dispersal agents in common use, CN is considered the most dangerous,[25] but exposure to CS or OC is not without risk. A recent systematic review examined data for 5131 people injured by crowd dispersal agents taken from 31 studies across 11 countries between 1990 and 2015.[24] The authors found 58 cases of permanent disability and 2 deaths associated with crowd dispersal agents, although most patients (98.7%) fully recovered. One death was caused by a traumatic brain injury from the impact of the chemical irritant munition, and the other caused by respiratory failure after CS aerosol was deployed inside a home.[24] In Hong Kong, a case report published in the wake of protests in 2020 described a photojournalist who, after repeated exposure to CS, presented with severe tracheobronchitis as well as contact dermatitis. However, after a 4-day hospital stay, he was much improved, and his pulmonary function tests were nearly back to normal at 6-week follow-up.[26]

The first step in crowd dispersal agent injury management is proper decontamination. Contaminated clothing should be removed and double-sealed in plastic bags, and the treating team should wear the proper PPE including gown, gloves, eye protection, and masks. Serious secondary injury to the treating team is unlikely, although minor effects, specifically eye lacrimation, can potentially incapacitate the treating team temporarily. As such, decontamination should occur in a well-ventilated space, removed from other patients, and while minimizing staff exposure.

Ocular symptoms are common and may include pain, decreased vision, or a foreign body sensation. Flushing with saline or water for 10–20 minutes is usually sufficient.[23] If significant symptoms persist consider corneal abrasion or the presence of a foreign body. The eye should be evaluated as with any other potential ocular emergency, with fluorescein stain and slit lamp exam. The mechanism of exposure (e.g., explosive or spray) should help establish pretest probability for mechanical injury on top of chemical injury. Repeated application of topical anesthetics can be useful to help patients tolerate the irrigation.

Most airway symptoms resolve after the patient is no longer exposed to the offending agent, especially after decontamination. The patients at highest risk for developing serious complications are those who experienced exposure to high concentrations in a confined space for extended periods of time and those with underlying pulmonary disease (primarily asthma and chronic obstructive pulmonary disease, COPD).[23] In general, management of these patients is similar to the management of any patient in respiratory distress, including close monitoring of oxygenation. Pulse oximetry is generally sufficient, but arterial blood gas can be sent if the pulse oximeter is unreliable, or the patient is ill appearing. Chest x-rays may be helpful to look for rare cases of pulmonary edema, although they are generally low yield. A portable chest x-ray and point-of-care ultrasound should be obtained in the unstable patient.

Dermatologic symptoms are also common following chemical irritant exposure. Even if patient is well appearing with no or minimal skin irritation after being thoroughly decontaminated, anticipatory guidance, and return precautions must be given, as symptoms can be delayed hours or even days from exposure.[27] Rarely, contact dermatitis may develop and should be managed with topical corticosteroids and antihistamines. Severe cases may warrant systemic steroids. In the rare case of a chemical burn from these agents, the management is the same as it would be for a thermal burn.[23]

Beyond immediate irritation and discomfort, emergency clinicians must also keep the secondary effects of crowd control agents in mind.[27] Even after decontamination, remnants of these agents can remain in a patient's oropharynx for hours to days. In a case report of a patient who required intubation for surgery 10 h after exposure to CS, marked laryngospasm made intubation difficult. Complicating the case still further, the anesthesiologist had to call on another physician because lacrimation from secondary exposure to the agent made it impossible for them to visualize the airway for the reintubation.[28]

Injury from Improvised Incendiary Devices

Although uncommon, improvised incendiary devices are also occasionally deployed during times of civil unrest, usually against public safety and law enforcement personnel. The most common of these devices is the so-called Molotov cocktail. The Molotov cocktail dates to 1939 during conflict between the Soviet Union and Finland, during which Finnish factories began making the devices in vodka bottles. Finnish troops used these "cocktails" against Soviet troops to great effect.[29] These devices are made of a glass bottle filled with gasoline, alcohol, or other flammable liquid. A cloth fuse is lit, and the device is thrown with the intent that the glass will break on impact and the fuel will ignite. Injuries include injuries from the vessel itself including lacerations, inhalation injury from smoke and other toxic fumes, and burns, which may be severe.

Management in the ED should follow basic principles of burn management. However, additional consideration should be given to potentially flammable contaminants on skin or clothing from unconsumed flammable material. Contaminated clothing should be promptly removed and secured. Removal of clothing is usually sufficient to remove material that could potentially off gas and ignite. However, the patient should be thoroughly decontaminated prior to any surgical management or other intervention that would involve electrocautery. Disposition should include the consideration of transfer to burn center, depending on the patient's injury burden.

Retinal Laser Injuries

Ocular trauma during civil unrest is typically secondary to trauma from projectiles. However, during several recent events lasers have been deployed with the intent of causing ocular injury to public safety and law enforcement personnel. During recent protests in Portland, OR the deputy director of the Department of Homeland Security reported that federal officers suffered 113 eye injuries.[30] While most cases of eye injury caused by commercially available lasers are self-limited, patients can present with symptoms ranging from eye discomfort to temporary blindness.

A laser is a device that emits an amplified optical light beam, and these devices are used in a wide variety of industrial, military, and civilian applications. Laser technology is increasingly available, and lasers are likewise increasingly more powerful. Damage can occur via photochemical, photomechanical, or photothermal mechanisms.[31] Photomechanical injuries occur through brief exposure to very high-power lasers, resulting in immediate tissue damage from the laser beam itself. Photochemical injuries occur with prolonged exposure to lower power light sources, such as solar light. Thermal injuries can occur with longer duration (microseconds to several seconds) to somewhat less powerful lasers. Heat from the laser beam causes protein coagulation and tissue damage. Injury caused by exposure to lasers depends on wavelength, exposure duration, spot size, power, and distance to source.

Following laser exposure, a patient may present with flashes or floaters, blepharospasm, tearing, or visual field deficits including blindness. Most laser eye injuries are painless, and discomfort is usually the result of self-inflicted corneal abrasions. Most patients will recall visualizing a light source, even when the light beam is outside of the visible spectrum.[31] The majority of symptoms are mild and self-limited, and almost all cases of discomfort or blindness are self-limited.

Any patient with a suspected eye injury due to laser exposure should have a thorough eye examination, as other causes of eye discomfort or vision changes are possible including exposure to irritants or orbital trauma. After ruling out ocular trauma, the patient should be referred to an ophthalmologist able to perform more advanced diagnostics.

Vignette 1 Conclusion

In this case, the community has time to prepare for arriving patients. An emergency clinician's priority should be to establish communication with local emergency medical services (EMS) and public safety to determine predicted crowd sizes and response capabilities. Given the reports of crowd dispersal agents and the warning of even larger numbers of protestors tonight, EMS agencies are staging vehicles and equipment far enough away – and at high elevations, if possible – to avoid contamination by crowd dispersal agents, yet also close enough to respond quickly. Emergency medical technicians and paramedics should also be prepared to don proper PPE.

Within the ED, coordinating other clinicians, nursing staff, and ancillary services to prepare for an influx of patients is paramount. To decompress the department, the larger community should also be warned to expect long wait times for routine care. All staff should be encouraged to review emergency preparedness plans including decontamination procedures.

The triage team should receive a few key reminders specific to assessing injuries sustained during civil unrest: (1) less-lethal projectiles can sometimes cause severe injury, especially if fired at close range; (2) treatment for exposure to crowd dispersal agents should begin in the decontamination area, with removal of clothing and copious flushing of eyes; (3) ocular exposure to chemical agents is generally not vision threatening unless the agent was dispersed as part of an explosive; and (4) the focus should be on those patients arriving with respiratory compromise, especially those with abnormal vital signs.

Vignette 2 Conclusion

Once patients begin to arrive, preparation yields dividends. The triage team is ready, wearing the proper PPE so they themselves do not become patients, and prepared to recognize potential life threats. Patients exposed to chemical agents are thoroughly decontaminated before evaluation, with clothes removed and double-bagged in plastic. If intubation is necessary, a back-up clinician should be aware, in case the procedure releases residual crowd control agent into the air and the primary airway clinician becomes incapacitated or has difficulty seeing due to lacrimation.

Patients with imminent airway compromise will take priority. A quick physical exam should help guide management of those with respiratory distress who appear stable: racemic epinephrine for upper airway symptoms (stridor), and albuterol and possibly steroids for those with wheezing, recognizing that life-threatening respiratory symptoms are rare in patients without underlying disease.

For those with traumatic injuries from projectiles, exam and history (including, importantly, knowledge of from what distance the projectile was fired, and what kind of projectile it was) will inform the imaging plan. For facial injuries, thin cuts obtained from a CT face can be helpful, and ocular exams are essential for patients with injuries from projectiles to the eye, with rapid decompression of retrobulbar hematoma with lateral canthotomy and cantholysis. Taser barbs are easy to remove – hold skin taut, pull out barb at a 90-degree angle. A small incision can be made, if needed. Tasers, even when discharged across the heart, are generally safe. These patients can usually wait for treatment.

Pro-Tips

- Establish good working relationships with local community leaders and law enforcement so you can get early notice if there is risk of civil unrest. This will give you time to mobilize additional resources and increase capacity at your hospital by moving or canceling elective care. Developing a response plan well in advance (including media/communication) is especially useful when unrest is not predicted and patients arrive at your department without warning.
- Law enforcement presence in the ED may be contentious. Limit law enforcement interaction with other patients unless necessary for patient care, patient and staff safety, or legal requirement.
- Attempt to separate patients with different viewpoints within the ED. As a healthcare provider, attempt to identify and limit any inherent bias and treat all patients with dignity and respect, regardless of political ideology. Documentation should remain neutral.
- If civil unrest is expected, or during planned demonstrations or other events in which civil unrest may develop, consider pre-deploying showers or other materials for decontamination of patients exposed to crowd dispersal agents. When dealing with crowd dispersal agents, clothing should be removed quickly and placed in a plastic bag. Decontamination should occur in a well-ventilated area to prevent secondary effects on staff or other patients.
- Barbs from conducted electrical weapons are usually straightforward to remove by holding skin taught and gently pulling at a 90-degree angle. Barbs lodged in the face, eye, or genitals may require specialist consultation.

References

1. U.S. Code Chapter 12 – Civil Disorders. Available from www.law.cornell.edu/uscod e/text/18/part-I/chapter-12.

2. Mitchell O. Understanding police use of force via hospital administrative data: prospects and problems. *JAMA Netw Open.* 2018;1(5):e182231.

3. Garner JH, Hickman MJ, Malega RW, Maxwell CD. Progress toward national estimates of police use of force. *PLoS One.* 2018;13(2):e0192932.

4. Lima J. Mass. General deployed hazmat tent to treat tear gas victims as protests turned violent. 2020; www.boston25news.com/new

s/local/mass-general-deployed-hazmat-tent-treat-tear-gas-victims-protests-turned-violent/5G4IR3DRYFB7PG52DDB4T4C DLM/. Accessed May 25, 2022.

5. Lee Jenkins J, Mason M. A Long Night in the emergency department during the Baltimore, Maryland (USA) riots. *Prehosp Disaster Med.* 2015;30(4):325–326.

6. Harada MY, Lara-Millan A, Chalwell LE. Policed patients: how the presence of law enforcement in the emergency department impacts medical care. *Ann Emerg Med.* 2021;78(6):738–748.

7. Law enforcement information gathering in the emergency department. *Ann Emerg Med.* 2017;70(6):942–943.

8. Strote J, Hickman MJ. Emergency department documentation of alleged police use of excessive force in cases where formal complaints are ultimately filed. *Am J Forensic Med Pathol.* 2018;39(4):309–311.

9. Bozeman WP, Stopyra JP, Klinger DA, Martin BP, Graham DD, Johnson 3rd JC, Mahoney-Tresoriero K, Vail SJ. Injuries associated with police use of force. *J Trauma Acute Care Surg.* 2018;84 (3):466–472.

10. Castillo EM, Prabhakar N, Luu B. Factors associated with law enforcement-related use-of-force injury. *Am J Emerg Med.* 2012;30(4):526–531.

11. Department of Justice, Office of Community Oriented Policing Services. *After-action assessment of the police response to the August 2014 demonstrations in Ferguson, Missouri.* Department of Justice, Office of Community Oriented Policing Services; 2015.

12. Haar RJ, Iacopino V, Ranadive N, Dandu M, Weiser SD. Death, injury and disability from kinetic impact projectiles in crowd-control settings: a systematic review. *BMJ Open.* 2017;7(12): e018154.

13. Kaske EA, Cramer SW, Pena Pino I, et al. Injuries from less-lethal weapons during the George Floyd Protests in Minneapolis. *N Engl J Med.* 2021;384(8):774–775.

14. Lartizien R, Schouman T, Raux M, Debelmas A, Lanciaux-Lemoine S,

Chauvin A, Toutee A, Touitou V, Bourges J-L, Goudot P, Bertolus C, Foy J-P. Yellow vests protests: facial injuries from rubber bullets. *Lancet.* 2019;394 (10197):469–470.

15. Brun PM, Bessereau J, Chenaitia H, Barberis C, Peyrol M. Commotio cordis as a result of neutralization shot with the Flash Ball less-lethal weapon. *Int J Cardiol.* 2012;158(3):e47–48.

16. Strasburger JF, Maron BJ. Commotio cordis. *N Engl J Med.* 2002;347(16):1248–1248.

17. Bleetman A, Steyn R, Lee C. Introduction of the Taser into British policing. Implications for UK emergency departments: an overview of electronic weaponry. *Emerg Med J.* 2004;21 (2):136–140.

18. Fish RM, Geddes LA. Effects of stun guns and tasers. *Lancet.* 2001;358 (9283):687–688.

19. Ordog GJ, Wasserberger J, Schlater T, Balasubramanium S. Electronic gun (Taser) injuries. *Ann Emerg Med.* 1987;16 (1):73–78.

20. MacDonald JM, Kaminski RJ, Smith MR. The effect of less-lethal weapons on injuries in police use-of-force events. *Am J Public Health.* 2009;99(12):2268–2274.

21. Bozeman WP, Teacher E, Winslow JE. Transcardiac conducted electrical weapon (TASER) probe deployments: incidence and outcomes. *J Emerg Med.* 2012;43 (6):970–975.

22. Vilke G, Chan T, Bozeman WP, Childers R. Emergency department evaluation after conducted energy weapon use: review of the literature for the clinician. *J Emerg Med.* 2019;57(5):740–746.

23. Schep LJ, Slaughter RJ, McBride DI. Riot control agents: the tear gases CN, CS and OC – A medical review. *J R Army Med Corps.* 2015;161(2):94–99.

24. Haar RJ, Iacopino V, Ranadive N, Weiser SD, Dandu M. Health impacts of chemical irritants used for crowd control: a systematic review of the injuries and deaths caused by tear gas and pepper spray. *BMC Public Health.* 2017;17(1):831.

25. Chapman AJ, White C. Death resulting from lacrimatory agents. *J Forensic Sci.* 1978;23(3):527–530.

26. Lam RPK, Wong KW, Wan CK. Allergic contact dermatitis and tracheobronchitis associated with repeated exposure to tear gas. *Lancet.* 2020;396(10247):e12.

27. Dimitroglou Y, Rachiotis G, Hadjichristodoulou C. Exposure to the riot control agent CS and potential health effects: a systematic review of the evidence. *Int J Environ Res Public Health.* 2015;12 (2):1397–1411.

28. Davey A, Moppett IK. Postoperative complications after CS spray exposure. *Anaesthesia.* 2004;59(12):1219–1220.

29. Stout J. The history of the Molotov cocktail, an iconic weapon of underdogs. *National Geographic* 2022.

30. Nelson S. Federal officers in Portland suffered 113 eye injuries from lasers, DHS official says. *New York Post.* 2020, August 4.

31. Mainster MA, Stuck BE, Brown J, Jr. Assessment of alleged retinal laser injuries. *Arch Ophthalmol.* 2004;122 (8):1210–1217.

Terrorism and Mass Casualty Incidents

Gregory R. Ciottone and Derrick Tin

Vignette

It's a beautiful Fall day in a New England City. An outdoor Oktoberfest gathering is taking place in the city park. As over 300 people gather to listen to music, eat sausages, and enjoy the weather, a drone is seen flying over the gathering. As people look up, some wave while others disregard and return their attention to the activities. Suddenly the drone releases what appears to be a mist of liquid from a reservoir located under its fuselage. People start to gasp and complain as many are doused by the liquid. Within several minutes people begin to drop to their knees and appear to lose consciousness. Some fall flat and show slowed breathing, while others become apneic. As this occurs people begin to scream and run from the scene in all directions. Some people run and then drop less than 100 yards away. The drone disappears and there is pandemonium at the scene.

911 is called and emergency medical services arrive on scene to find more than 100 people down with no obvious signs of trauma. They call for multiple ambulances and relay to central dispatch that there has been a mass casualty incident (MCI). They then begin to triage and attend to patients with life-threatening conditions. Notification is made to your emergency department (ED) to expect 10–13 patients.

- What toxidrome(s) are considered based on the information provided?
- What preparations should be made in the ED?

Introduction

Terrorism is a complex, multidimensional phenomenon and an often-contested concept, with many varying national and regional definitions and no universally accepted legal definition, making research in this field particularly challenging.[1,2] From a healthcare perspective, however, the subtle nuances in defining terrorism matter less in terms of medical preparation, education, and response: all intentional, man-made, mass casualty events will share a degree of commonality and the recently created field of Counter-Terrorism Medicine (CTM) remains focused on analyzing and researching the healthcare impacts of such events.[3] Over the past decade the world has witnessed an increase in sophisticated, asymmetric, multimodality terrorist attacks,[4] peaking in 2014 with over 16,000 documented events[5] around the world in that year alone. Although attacks globally have been trending downward since that peak, particularly in the past 2 years during the coronavirus disease 2019 (COVID-19) pandemic when opportunities for mass gatherings (and hence potential targets) were limited and travel logistics significantly affected, counter-terrorism and intelligence analysts have seen a dramatic rise in domestic extremist activity in recent times.[6] The COVID-19 pandemic and widespread misinformation have ignited feelings of mistrust toward medical sectors and displeasure at governmental mandates, giving an opportunity to fringe extremist and terrorist organizations to recruit, infiltrate, and plan attacks on western soil.

In the past, terrorist events were often linear, consisting of a single bombing or ballistic attack that, once resolved, was the extent of the incident. Today's extremist groups have easier access to sophisticated technologies that can be easily adapted to cause mass harm. Off-the-shelf drones can be easily modified to deliver chemical weapons, cyberattacks on healthcare systems have been shown to be detrimental to patient outcomes, and three-dimensional printing of firearms bypasses the safety barriers of background checks. For urban EDs, which are also potential targets for a primary terrorist attack,[7] this represents a gathering storm necessitating focused, proactive steps to enhance preparedness.

Mass Casualty Incidents

Mass casualty incidents (MCI) are sudden, unpredictable events that always involve some degree of patient surge that can strain ED and hospital resources. The Las Vegas shooting in 2017 resulted in more than 600 casualties presenting to local hospitals, many of whom had military-grade gunshot wounds.[8] Hospitals have long had difficulty rapidly pivoting from daily operations to mass casualty care when a sudden event occurs.[9] Out of financial necessity, hospitals today are run extremely efficiently, with virtually no inherent surge capacity in the event of the influx of a large number of critical patients. This means that EDs must develop emergency operations plans that allow for increased surge capacity when required by events such as MCIs. In addition, because injury patterns can differ and are often more severe in MCI, particularly terrorist events, putting further strain on ED resources, EDs should also regularly update staff in current trauma care. While ballistic and blast injuries have long been major components of terrorism-related MCI, with the advent of unique modalities such as cars and trucks in vehicle ramming attacks and the use of military-grade ballistic weapons, traumatic mass casualties from an MCI can have a combination of blunt, penetrating, and burn injuries. Injury patterns seen in MCI may be unfamiliar to civilian emergency physicians, as some wound patterns will be similar to battlefield injuries. Because historical data have shown that targeted terrorist attacks result in higher acuity injuries and more utilization of hospital resources,[10] when notification is given that an ED will be receiving incoming patients from an MCI it is important to understand whether it is an intentional or accidental event. As an example, an intentional bombing is much different from an accidental explosion. While in both cases the ED must prepare for the arrival of multiple traumatic casualties, due to deliberate targeting there will be more critical injuries and higher utilization of resources when they are coming from an intentional attack.

The capability of an ED to handle MCI is largely determined by patient surge capacity, which can be enhanced by disaster response actions such as reverse triage that create space to receive patients quickly. Reverse triage rapidly empties an ED by discharging appropriate patients for outpatient work-up and treatment, and sending stable patients who are awaiting admission or whose work-up is nearly complete to inpatient wards.[11] This allows capacity to be quickly increased upon notification of an MCI. Other preparedness steps include enhancing the efficiency of laboratory and radiology services and providing training to staff in the care of victims of non-conventional modalities, such as chemical, biological, radiological, nuclear, and high-yield explosives (CBRNE).

Chemical, Biological, Radiological, Nuclear, or High-Yield Explosives

Use of modalities such as CBRNE in terrorist attack is of growing concern. Between 2012 and 2021, the more frequent use of chemical warfare agents (CWA) on civilian targets in conflict zones, including chlorine and sarin in Syria,[12] and assassination attempts utilizing VX[13] and Novichok[14,15] in Malaysia, Russia, and the United Kingdom, demonstrates an increased availability of these potential weapons of mass destruction. In addition, the United States continues to suffer from a significant opioid crisis, and drug overdose deaths remain a leading cause of death, despite efforts to curb the influx of fentanyl derivatives onto the streets of America. While the opioid crisis is tragic in and of itself, it also raises a clear national security issue: The increasing availability of dangerous potential chemical weapons in the form of fentanyl and its derivatives like carfentanil, which is significantly more potent.[16]

This ease of access and increased emergence of potential chemical weapons into our communities means that urban EDs must be ready to respond in the event of a chemical attack mass casualty. While military countermeasures have been developed and practiced, civilian EDs are largely unprepared for any form of CBRNE attack, particularly one utilizing CWA.[17] Early identification of agent class, availability of antidotes, including the enormous amounts of atropine or naloxone that would be required in a mass casualty nerve agent and opioid attack, respectively, remain operational and logistical concerns. The recent development of a field triage protocol for the classes of CWA most likely to be sourced and used in terrorist attacks is a step toward improving civilian preparedness[18] (Figure 14.1). However, more attention to response training, stockpiling antidotes, streamlining decontamination capabilities, and maximizing surge capacity are required. The Moscow theater attack (where aerosolized fentanyl derivatives and halothane were the most likely agents used) resulted in 117 deaths, largely due to delays in recognising the mechanism and causal agents of the injuries, as well as logistical challenges of getting antidote to the large numbers of casualties.[19] Historically, chemical attacks have occurred predominantly in high population density settings, making it a preparedness concern for urban EDs.

For similar ease of accessibility reasons, an intentional radiological event is also of concern.[20] While a thermonuclear detonation is highly unlikely, yet regrettably possible, a radiological dispersal device (RDD) consisting of conventional explosives dispersing radioactive material, often referred to as a "dirty bomb," is a more likely scenario. The world witnessed the potentially devastating effects of a RDD when Chernobyl caught fire and exploded in 1986, propelling 50 million curies (Ci) of xenon, 40 million Ci of iodine-131, and 3 million Ci of cesium-137 into the atmosphere that was detected as far north as Sweden.[21] The Chernobyl disaster, with the resultant "Exclusion Zone" that is 30 km in diameter and uninhabitable for 30 years, was the world's first dirty bomb, albeit an accidental one, and demonstrated the potentially catastrophic effects of such an event. A common misperception is that terrorist organizations would have to source, transport, and then utilize a radioactive source to successfully detonate an RDD. This is not the case; there are ample sources available in the community. All hospital and healthcare facilities with radiology capabilities have such radiological material. An intentional attack on a healthcare radiology department could be considered an RDD. In addition, most smoke detectors contain americium-241, an alpha-emitting radioactive isotope, which could also be stockpiled and used in an RDD.[22] Emergency department preparation for some form of radiological attack should consist first of a high index of suspicion so that radiation can be

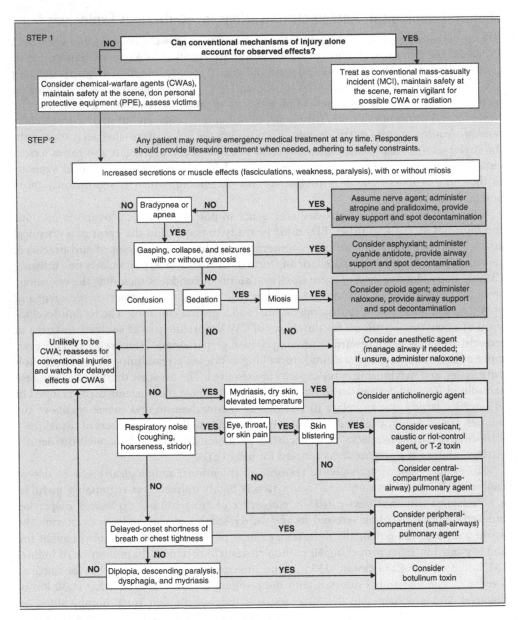

Figure 14.1 Field triage algorithm for acute-phase chemical weapons attack
Source: Ciottone GR. Toxidrome recognition in chemical-weapons attacks. *N Engl J Med*. 2018;378(17):1611–1620. doi: 10.1056/NEJMra1705224. PMID: 29694809.

detected. This would hopefully happen at the scene. Following such an attack, radiological decontamination, both external and internal if needed, should be done and steps to determine the approximate dose equivalent of victims and responders in Roentgen equivalent man (REM) understood. This will allow a prediction of the degree, if any, of acute radiation syndrome (ARS) victims may have, and will drive their treatment going forward. ARS occurs in four phases: prodromal, latency, illness manifestation, and recovery. Treatment is largely supportive and includes the use of anti-emetics and hematopoietic agents.[23]

While bioterrorism remains rare,[24] the COVID-19 pandemic has exposed a number of critical flaws in the biosecurity arrangements of many countries, and with the advent of clustered regularly interspaced short palindromic repeats (CRISPR) technologies, a man-made intentional bio-attack is not out of the realm of near-future possibilities. Unless a biotoxin is used, which would mimic a chemical weapon attack in many ways, a bio-attack may have an insidious onset and require astute clinicians to detect in the early phases. The "Amerithrax" attacks in the Fall of 2021 may have continued longer undetected and killed many more had not an astute physician suspected anthrax in one of his patients coming thorough the ED on October 2, 2001 in Palm Beach County, FL.[25] Once a bio-attack is detected, management will be dependent on both hospital capacity and a robust public health system, as witnessed during the COVID-19 pandemic. While not a short-term mass casualty response, urban EDs may have to cope with patient surge over weeks to months and, with their daily large volume of patients and higher likelihood of being in the epicenter of a bio-attack, are ideally situated to conduct bio-surveillance for early detection.

Counter-Terrorism Medicine

Given these unique threats and due to the increase in asymmetric, multimodality attacks, often involving either primary or secondary attacks on healthcare,[7] along with the significant psychosocial and financial impact of terrorist attacks on victims and affected communities, CTM was recently established as a sub-specialty of Disaster Medicine.[3] CTM addresses the mitigation, preparedness, and response to these attacks on civilian populations in an attempt to match the sophistication put into the planning and execution of attacks with equal sophistication in responding to them. The clarification must always be made that CTM only addresses the healthcare implications to terrorist attacks. CTM is never to include counter-terrorism activities such as prevention, intelligence, or armed response. However, CTM does give healthcare a seat at the counter-terrorism table, so as to better integrate medical response into the overall mission.

Concerning preparedness, in an analysis of the 2001 terrorist attacks in the United States, the 9/11 commission determined "The most important failure was one of imagination. We do not believe leaders understood the gravity of the threat."[26] As part of the solution to this very sobering finding that supports the need for its creation, CTM was established as a healthcare counter-measure to the "imagination" of those intending to do harm. The healthcare response to terrorist events now must have the capability and capacity to care for hundreds or more patients suffering from complex injury patterns that may be a result of any combination of blast, vehicle ramming, military ballistics, melee, or CBRNE modalities, in the context of unique potential delivery platforms and strategies, such as drone swarm chemical release over mass gatherings. CTM aims to address and remedy the preparedness and response shortfalls for such complex attack scenarios, and enable the healthcare sector to be better prepared.

Where Does Counter-Terrorism Medicine Sit?

There has been some discussion concerning the medical response to terrorism over the past 50 years, including some healthcare-rooted initiatives to address the issue.[27-29] CTM has evolved out of a number of them to include the increasing complexity of attacks, and the subsequent need for more thorough, imaginative preparedness and response strategies. One of the topics of discussion is where CTM fits in today's environment of operations-based medicine, and what events should its practice include. While there are clear lines of distinction between mass casualty-producing events like hybrid warfare, lone-wolf attacks, and state-sponsored attacks on civilians with terrorist attack, for the purposes of the healthcare response, those lines can be blurred. CTM encompasses any form of strategic attack on civilians that results in mass casualties. Court *et al.* set the parameters of what should be included in the practice of CTM as "Intent, Violence, and Healthcare Impact,"[3] and that it should have shared competencies with a number of related fields (Figure 14.2). By addressing the practice of CTM in this manner, healthcare is freed to concern itself more with the medical needs, and less with the ideological and political nuances.

In addition, rather than create silos in medicine to address these different but related threats, CTM seeks to develop the necessary competencies, and to bring into the initiative those medical specialties required to address the unique low-frequency, high-acuity nature of terrorism. Healthcare must treat this gathering storm in the same manner it does all other public health crises.

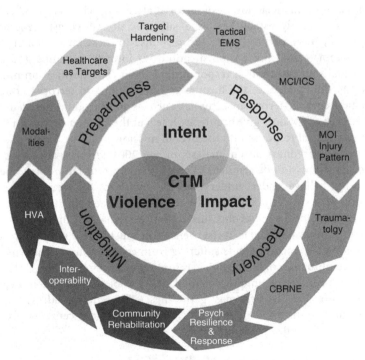

Figure 14.2 The parameters and relationships of Counter-Terrorism Medicine
Source: Court M, Edwards B, Issa F, Voskanyan A, Ciottone G. Counter-Terrorism Medicine: Creating a medical initiative mandated by escalating asymmetric attacks. *Prehosp Disaster Med.* 2020;35(6):595–598. doi: 10.1017/S1049023X2000103X. Epub 2020 Aug 14. PMID: 32792026.

The Practice of Counter-Terrorism Medicine

There is concern that the recent surge in asymmetric attacks on major cities, mass gatherings, and transportation hubs will, after the brief lull during COVID-19, again begin to escalate.[30] These attacks, and their exploitation of the multitude of vulnerabilities that are present today, can be considered a growing public health crisis. As we inadvertently present "soft" targets through our very open societies, terrorists will continue to attack us in ways designed to maximize casualties. Healthcare responders and hospitals are and will be on the forefront of caring for these patients. In order to be most effective, while also protecting the safety of personnel, certain counter-terrorism medicine steps must be learned, understood, and implemented.

In order to develop a healthcare strategy for terrorist events a hospital must first take steps toward optimizing its response to a MCI. Most large medical centers today will have a department of emergency management, which directs efforts to prepare the hospital for both internal and external disaster events, including MCI. Often times, an emergency physician will serve as either the Director or Medical Director of this department. Many of the emergency preparedness steps taken are designed to improve throughput, such as optimization of diagnostic systems, increasing efficiency and training of the workforce, space optimization, and asset realignment to address changing needs. Hospital-based emergency managers will also conduct hazard vulnerability analyses, and use that risk stratification exercise to design emergency operations plans (EOP). Such plans outline the appropriate response of all hospital departments, services, and personnel in the event of an MCI or disaster. While the process of creating an EOP is a good exercise to do, the EOP itself should not be counted on solely to manage an MCI. Many disaster events will take unanticipated changes in course and these cascading compound disasters will likely create scenarios unaccounted for by even the most extensive of EOPs, prompting the need to deviate from and modify the planned response.[31] The planning process that goes into the creation of an EOP, however, is a valuable step toward preparedness. Better the planning than the plan.

MCI preparedness requires the ED to operate efficiently, triage effectively, and integrate with other services like surgery, intensive care, and radiology smoothly. Intentional events, such as terrorist attacks, have been shown to cause higher injury severity scores, utilize more hospital resources, and require implementation of disaster triage strategies.[10] As discussed, in this case, surge capacity strategies such as disaster triage and "reverse triage"[32] should be developed and exercised. Handling surge from mass casualty incidents is a hospital-wide effort sometimes requiring realignment of personnel and resources. When exercised, attention should be paid to challenging systems not commonly accustomed to handling surge, as the ED is, but rather parts of the hospital that are not. Reverse triage drills do exactly that; test the ability of inpatient wards to accept an influx of stable but partially worked-up patients from the ED, so that the ED can then increase its capacity to handle the incoming surge.

In the event of a terrorist attack, surge on the healthcare system can be expected, but there are other considerations as well. Clinical unfamiliarity to terrorist attack modalities is a concern for clinicians. Trauma presentations may be different with hospital clinicians potentially dealing with unfamiliar complex injury patterns. Vehicle ramming attacks differ from accidental vehicular crashes, for example, as the perpetrator in the former will often accelerate rather than decelerate toward victims, and may intentionally run over those already injured. Perpetrators may inflict further harm to an already injured victim using a different modality such as bladed weapons or firearms as they abandon their vehicles and continue their attack rampage, as seen during the London Bridge attacks in 2017. The treatment of victims of suicide attacks also necessitate special bio-prophylaxis considerations as a result of implantation of biological remains, and while blast injuries are well documented in medical literature, high-explosive load blasts with irregular secondary complex shrapnel injuries remain relatively rare in frequency outside of conflict zones. The lack of exposure to such attack modalities could result in unfamiliarity and delayed interventions; therefore, one of the primary purposes of CTM is to centralize and provide the best evidence-based management of such low-frequency, high-acuity injuries to civilian clinicians. Furthermore, responding to a mass casualty terrorist event adds a significant and unique mental health burden on clinician responders. Medical organizations and systems need to have psychological preparedness and response strategies in place to ensure staff well-being and safety, as well as continuity of care in the aftermath.

Healthcare as a Target

While secondary attacks on healthcare in the prehospital setting have been occurring for decades, intentionally targeting healthcare personnel and facilities have recently emerged as a concerning terrorist tactic around the world. CTM specifically discusses the merits of hardening soft structures such as medical facilities and ambulances as a risk-mitigation strategy to ensure the ongoing provision of medical services in the face of direct threats.[33] While medical first responders were once only expected to operate exclusively in a cold zone environment, the changing world of threat has increasing requirements and expectations for medical operations within the hot and warm zones, and CTM has incorporated many of the lessons learned in tactical medicine (such as tactical emergency casualty care) into its curriculum.

The practice of CTM should involve a cross-silo approach that focuses healthcare preparedness and response on these intentionally designed high-acuity, low-frequency events.[3] Research to date around CTM has seen disaster medicine specialists collaborate with criminologists, tactical medicine specialists, experts in unconventional weapons and various law enforcement and security experts to bridge these silos that currently exist. Field CTM response extends into the ED, with the same principles required in the response to terrorism.

Summary

Urban EDs play a significant role in the care of victims from MCI. While many are accidental, intentional attacks pose unique scenarios requiring a heightened level of preparedness and response. The intentionality of terrorist incidents, along with the sophistication in planning that may include primary attack on healthcare assets, demand that emergency physicians and EDs address these as uniquely complex events requiring increased vigilance in planning.

Vignette Conclusion

The responders find the predominant toxidrome is sedation, bradypnea/apnea, and miosis. An opioid is suspected based on the toxidrome. Multiple ambulances arrive on scenes and as responders treat the patients with naloxone and bag valve mask (BVM), some become symptomatic themselves with mild sedation and bradypnea. Area hospitals are notified and a call goes out to deliver as much naloxone and BVMs to the scene as possible. Patients begin to be transported by ambulance and personal vehicles to area EDs, which become inundated with opioid-exposed patients. Naloxone stores are exhausted across the city. Despite best efforts, 130 event attendees and 3 responders die as a result of this carfentanyl attack via drone.

Pro-Tips

- With the over-abundance of fentanyl and its derivatives, now so readily available in civilian settings due to the ongoing opioid crisis, we must prepare for the possibility of opioid attack via drone or some other delivery mechanism.
- When faced with mass casualties with no obvious conventional trauma source, a chemical attack must be considered.
- Scene safety in terrorist events include both conventional hazards and the possibility of the scene still being active.
- Stores of traditional antidotes like naloxone for opioid attack and atropine for nerve agent attack in a mass casualty situation can be rapidly depleted. Contingency plans for sourcing such counter-measures should be established as part of hospital preparedness.
- The 911 Commission stated one of the biggest failures that led to the attacks of September 11, 2001 was lack of imagination in mitigation and preparedness. Counter-Terrorism Medicine seeks to be more proactive in the healthcare response to terrorism.

References

1. United Nations Office on Drugs and Crime. Defining Terrorism. Available at: www.unodc.org/e4j/en/terrorism/module-4/key-issues/defining-terrorism.html. Accessed April 6, 2022.

2. Schmid AP. *The Routledge Handbook of Terrorism Research*. Routledge, 2011; 50–60, 86–87.

3. Court M, Edwards B, Issa F, Voskanyan A, Ciottone G. Counter-Terrorism Medicine: creating a medical initiative mandated by escalating asymmetric attacks. *Prehosp Disaster Med*. 2020;35(6):595–598. doi: 10.1017/S1049023X2000103X. PMID: 32792026.

4. Tin D, Margus C, Ciottone GR. Half-a-century of terrorist attacks: weapons selection, casualty outcomes, and implications for counter-terrorism medicine. *Prehosp Disaster Med*. 2021;36 (5):526–530. doi: 10.1017/S1049023X21000868. PMID: 34392864.

5. Ritchie H, Hasell J, Appel C, Roser M. Terrorism. Our World in Data. 2019 Available at: https://ourworldindata.org/terrorism. Accessed April 6, 2022.

6. National Strategy for Countering Domestic Terrorism. 2021. Available at: www.whitehouse.gov/wp-content/uploads/2021/06/National-Strategy-for-Countering-Domestic-Terrorism.pdf. Accessed May 19, 2022.

7. Cavaliere GA, Alfalasi R, Jasani GN, Ciottone GR, Lawner BJ. Terrorist attacks against healthcare facilities: a review. *Health Secur*. 2021;19(5):546–550. doi: 10.1089/hs.2021.0004. PMID: 34319798.

8. Lozada MJ, Cai S, Li M, Davidson SL, Nix J, Ramsey G. The Las Vegas mass shooting: an analysis of blood component administration and blood bank donations. *J Trauma Acute Care Surg*. 2019;86 (1):128–133. doi: 10.1097/TA.0000000000002089. PMID: 30371625.

9. Marcozzi DE, Pietrobon R, Lawler JV, French MT, Mecher C, Peffer J, Baehr NE, Browne BJ. Development of a Hospital Medical Surge Preparedness Index using a national hospital survey. *Health Serv Outcomes Res Method.* 2020;20:60–83. https://doi.org/10.1007/s10742-020-00208-6.

10. Kosashvili Y, Aharonson-Daniel L, Peleg K, Horowitz A, Laor D, Blumenfeld A. Israeli hospital preparedness for terrorism-related multiple casualty incidents: can the surge capacity and injury severity distribution be better predicted? *Injury.* 2009;40(7):727–731. doi: 10.1016/j. injury.2008.11.010. Erratum in: *Injury.* 2010;41(7):1076. PMID: 19394934.

11. Pollaris G, Sabbe M. Reverse triage: more than just another method. *Eur J Emerg Med.* 2016;23(4):240–247. doi: 10.1097/MEJ.0000000000000339. PMID: 26479736.

12. Brooks J, Erickson TB, Kayden S, Ruiz R, Wilkinson S, Burkle FM Jr. Responding to chemical weapons violations in Syria: legal, health, and humanitarian recommendations. *Confl Health.* 2018;12:12. doi: 10.1186/s13031-018-0143-3. PMID: 29479374; PMCID: PMC5817898.

13. Kim Jong-nam killing: 'VX nerve agent' found on his face. BBC. 2017. Available at: www.bbc.com/news/world-asia-39073389. Accessed April 6, 2022.

14. Vale JA, Marrs TC, Maynard RL. Novichok: a murderous nerve agent attack in the UK. *Clin Toxicol (Phila).* 2018;56(11):1093–1097. doi: 10.1080/15563650.2018.1469759. PMID: 29757015.

15. Greathouse B, Zahra F, Brady MF. Acetylcholinesterase inhibitors toxicity. In: StatPearls [Internet]. StatPearls Publishing, 2022. PMID: 30571049.

16. Negri A, Townshend H, McSweeney T, Angelopoulou O, Banayoti H, Prilutskaya M, Bowden-Jones O, Corazza O. Carfentanil on the darknet: potential scam or alarming public health threat? *Int J Drug Policy.* 2021;91:103118.

doi: 10.1016/j.drugpo.2021.103118. PMID: 33482605.

17. Razak S, Hignett S, Barnes J. Emergency department response to chemical, biological, radiological, nuclear, and explosive events: a systematic review. *Prehosp Disaster Med.* 2018;33(5):543–549. doi: 10.1017/S1049023X18000900. PMID: 30379127.

18. Ciottone GR. Toxidrome recognition in chemical-weapons attacks. *N Engl J Med.* 2018;378(17):1611–1620. doi: 10.1056/NEJMra1705224. PMID: 29694809.

19. Wax PM, Becker CE, Curry SC. Unexpected "gas" casualties in Moscow: a medical toxicology perspective. *Ann Emerg Med.* 2003;41(5):700–5. doi: 10.1067/mem.2003.148.

20. United Nations Office of Counter-Terrorism. Chemical, biological, radiological and nuclear terrorism. Available at: www.un.org/counterterrorism/cct/chemical-biological-radiological-and-nuclear-terrorism. Accessed April 6, 2022.

21. Bonte FJ. Chernobyl retrospective. *Semin Nucl Med.* 1988;18(1):16–24. doi:10.1016/s0001-2998(88)80016-3. PMID: 3278382.

22. United States Nuclear Regulatory Commission, January 7, 2021. Available at: www.nrc.gov/reading-rm/doc-collections/fact-sheets/smoke-detectors.html. Accessed April 6, 2022.

23. Radiation Emergency Medical Management, US Department of Health and Human Services. February 17, 2022. Available at: https://remm.hhs.gov/ars.htm. Accessed April 6, 2022.

24. Tin D, Sabeti P, Ciottone GR. Bioterrorism: an analysis of biological agents used in terrorist events. *Am J Emerg Med.* 2022;54:117–121. doi: 10.1016/j.ajem.2022.01.056. PMID: 35152120; PMCID: PMC8818129.

25. Bush LM, Perez MT. The anthrax attacks 10 years later. *Ann Intern Med.* 2012;156(1 Pt 1):41–44. doi: 10.7326/0003-4819-155-12-201112200-00373. PMID: 21969275.

26. *9/11 Commission Report*. 2004. Available at: www.govinfo.gov/content/pkg/GPO-911R EPORT/pdf/GPO-911REPORT-24.pdf. Accessed April 29, 2022.

27. Cole LA. Raising awareness about terror medicine. *Clin Dermatol*. 2011;29 (1):100–102. doi: 10.1016/j. clindermatol.2010.07.015. PMID: 21146738.

28. Psychiatrists and terrorism. *Can Med Assoc J*. 1976;115(8):797. PMID: 987843; PMCID: PMC1878835.

29. Rignault DP. Recent progress in surgery for the victims of disaster, terrorism, and war – introduction. *World J Surg*. 1992;16 (5):885–887. doi: 10.1007/BF02066986. PMID: 1462624.

30. Tin D, Hertelendy AJ, Hart A, Ciottone GR. 50 Years of mass-fatality terrorist attacks: a retrospective study of target demographics, modalities, and injury patterns to better inform future counter-terrorism medicine preparedness and response. *Prehosp Disaster Med*. 2021;36(5):531–535. doi: 10.1017/ S1049023X21000819. PMID: 34369349.

31. Tin D, Hart A, Ciottone G. Rethinking disaster vulnerabilities. *Am J Emerg Med*. 2020:S0735-6757(20)30973-6. doi: 10.1016/j.ajem.2020.10.073.

32. Pollaris G, Sabbe M. Reverse triage: more than just another method. *Eur J Emerg Med*. 2016;23(4):240–247. doi: 10.1097/ MEJ.0000000000000339. PMID: 26479736.

33. Tin D, Hart A, Ciottone GR. Hardening hospital defences as a counter-terrorism medicine measure. *Am J Emerg Med*. 2021;45:667–668. doi: 10.1016/j. ajem.2020.10.051. PMID: 33153832.

Chapter 15

Overcrowding, Triage, and Care Rationing

Samita M. Heslin and Peter Viccellio

Vignette 1

The Medical Director of an urban emergency department (ED) has solicited help in improving ED overcrowding and boarding. This ED has nearly 100,000 patient visits annually, is a Level-1 trauma center, a comprehensive stroke center, and a STEMI center. This ED is also part of a 500-bed hospital that offers a full-range of medical specialty care, including hospitalist medicine, internal medicine and pediatrics medicine subspecialties (i.e., cardiology, nephrology, gastroenterology, rheumatology, hematology/oncology, infectious disease, and pulmonary, and critical care), obstetrics and gynecology, and surgical subspecialties (i.e., general surgery, neurosurgery, pediatric surgery, surgical oncology, trauma surgery).

Over the last year, this urban ED has been facing the following problems.

Boarding: After ED patients are admitted to an inpatient service, there are frequently no open beds available in the hospital for the patients to go to. Although the ED has 70 beds, given an average of 30 boarders, the ED effectively has 40 beds for new patients. These boarded patients are cared for by ED nurses and other ED staff members. Because these patients need ED staff and ED beds/space while boarding in the ED, this delays the care of new ED patients who need to be seen from the waiting room.

Overcrowding: The ED faces overcrowding problems due to both the influx of new ED patients as well as the boarding of admitted patients. Because there are more patients than rooms in the ED, there are also many patients in the ED hallways.

- What are the causes of ED overcrowding and boarding?
- What are hospital-level solutions for ED overcrowding and boarding?

Vignette 2

In addition, the ED mentioned in Clinical Vignette 1 is facing increased wait times for patients to see an ED clinician. Although patients are triaged by a nurse immediately after they arrive in the ED, patients often have to wait several hours to be seen by a physician during the peak ED hours. The ED medical director has asked for help improving ED triage during these peak hours.

- How can traditional ED triage be modified to better care for patients in overcrowded EDs?
- What are Emergency Department-level solutions for ED overcrowding and boarding?

Introduction

Emergency Department Overcrowding and Boarding

There were over 130 million ED visits in 2018 in the United States, of which 20 million were admitted to the hospital.[1] Between 40% and 50% of all EDs in the United States and two thirds of metropolitan EDs report that they experience crowding problems.[2] Metropolitan EDs in particular are affected due to small footprints relative to the number of patients in their service area. Hospitals often operate at or over census, which directly impacts the care of patients in the ED. The lack of hospital capacity leads to ED overcrowding due to boarding of admitted patients in the ED, which limits ED space, overwhelms ED staff, increases ED wait times, and decreases ED throughput.

Emergency department overcrowding and boarding have a detrimental impact on patient care and patient safety[3]:

- Emergency department overcrowding increases total hospital length of stay (LOS) by 1–3 days.[4]
- Emergency department overcrowding increases the number of patients that leave the ED without being seen, many of whom have serious conditions that warrant inpatient admission.[5]
- There are many resulting patient care concerns – ED overcrowding has been shown to delay imaging of stroke patients, administration of antibiotics for pneumonia, care of long bone fractures in children, and administration of pain medication for adults.[6–9]
- Due to ED overcrowding, only 67% of acutely ill patients are seen within recommended times[10] and 10% of critical patients wait more than an hour to see a physician.[11,12]
- Patients with acute coronary symptom (ACS) experience an increased complication rate during crowded times.[13]
- Emergency department boarding increases 10- and 30-day mortality rates.[14–16]

There are several interventions, largely ineffective, that have been proposed to solve the ED overcrowding problem. Interventions that divert non-urgent patients have not shown to improve flow and some of these patients will require admission to the hospital.[17,18] Ambulance diversion does not improve boarding. Additionally, interventions that target expanding ED capacity by increasing ED space or hiring more ED staff may not have a long-term impact because they likely will result in increasing the ED capacity to hold admitted patients rather than improving ED flow and throughput.

Hospital-Level Solutions

There are several possible solutions to ED overcrowding and boarding. Together, these interventions can improve hospital capacity and decrease ED boarding.

Smoothing Elective Admissions

Because admissions through the ED are generally uncontrollable and unschedulable, they can fluctuate on a daily basis. On Mondays and Tuesdays, there is generally an increased number of patients being admitted through the ED – some patients may have waited until the beginning of the week to see their outpatient physician and were sent in for further evaluation in the ED. However, ED admissions are overall steady state during the weekdays. Elective admissions are schedulable and thus controllable. Most elective admissions are generally in the beginning of the week (i.e., Mondays and Tuesdays), particularly surgical elective admissions. There are many reasons for this phenomenon, including historical preferences and scheduling practices[19] as well as decreased preoperative and postoperative services on the weekends. Due to the increased elective admissions in the beginning of the week, this results in artificial variability in hospital flow and significantly impacts hospital capacity. Because elective admissions compete directly with ED admissions for inpatient floor and intensive care unit (ICU) beds, this results in ED boarding and overcrowding.

Smoothing elective admissions, so that elective admissions are equally distributed across the week, can improve hospital capacity.[20] Smoothing can help with predicting staff numbers and assist with bed assignments. When Cincinnati Children's Hospital smoothed elective admissions, they cut wait times by 30% and increased revenue by $137 million.[21]

Early Discharge

Emergency department admissions increase throughout the day, as ED volume increases. If ED-admitted patients do not have an inpatient bed, they board in the ED as admitted patients. This can impact the ability to see new patients in the ED because there is a finite amount of space and number of staff in the ED. Discharging inpatients earlier in the day can help open inpatient beds for patients admitted thorough the ED. This would involve early initiation of tests and ancillary services, such as physical therapy, social work and case management services, and consults. When NYU-Langone Medical Center launched a Discharge Before Noon initiative, they were able to increase their rate of discharges before noon from 5% to 42% in five years without increasing readmission rates.[22]

Weekend Discharge

There is a significant variability in discharges on the weekends compared to the weekdays. The New York State Statewide Planning and Research Cooperative System (SPARCS) database shows that on the weekends, there are dramatically fewer discharges than on weekdays and the length of stay is shorter for patients discharged on Saturday compared to Monday. There may be many reasons why patients are not discharged on the weekends, including lack of services (i.e., radiological imaging, ECHOs, Physical Therapy, Occupational Therapy, Social Services); inability of certain outpatient facilities to accept discharged patients (i.e., rehabilitation centers, assisted-living facilities, nursing homes); and certain tests needed for discharge may not be performed on the weekends. Hospitals should evaluate what are the stopgaps to weekend discharges in their facilities and create initiatives to improve access to these services on the weekends.

Full Capacity Action Plan/Full Capacity Protocol – When All Else Fails

When hospital capacity is exhausted, the Full Capacity Protocol (FCP) can help decrease the number of patients boarding in the ED by moving these patients to inpatient units. Under the FCP, these patients would be redistributed to spaces available in the inpatient units, such as hallways, exam rooms, and conference rooms. Intensive Care patients would continue to stay in the ED until an ICU or step-down unit bed becomes available. The FCP has been shown to decrease ED boarding, improve ED wait times, shorten overall length of stay, and improve patient satisfaction.[23-27]

Emergency Department–Level Solutions

Traditionally, ED triage is completed by a nurse, who briefly evaluates the patient and assigns an Emergency Severity Index (ESI). In overcrowded EDs, additional triage methods might help improve patient care. However, these triage methods do not solve the inherent issues that cause ED overcrowding, such as the lack of hospital capacity as discussed in the above section.

Team Triage is a form of triage conducted by a group of clinicians (often a nurse, advanced practice provider, and/or physician). Although there are many versions of Team Triage, generally it entails a brief evaluation by the team including vitals, assignment of an ESI, ordering of basic laboratory orders, ordering of some radiological studies, and placement of an IV. During Team Triage, patients may also receive some medications such as anti-emetics, antipyretics, and pain medications. After the Team Triage process, the patient will often return to a waiting area until a room/spot opens for further evaluation in the main zones of the ED, which might be a few hours in overcrowded EDs. While the patient is in the waiting area, however, their blood tests may result and they may have some of their radiological imaging performed. Additionally, ED staff will be alerted to any critical results from the laboratory or radiological testing, which will help identify any patients that need to be immediately evaluated. Team Triage has also been shown to decrease time to discharge but not lead to increased testing.[28] Without Team Triage, these patients may have to wait hours to be placed in an ED room/spot and then have their workup (i.e., laboratory orders, IVs, radiological orders) started. However, Team Triage can be an expensive process because several clinicians will need to be part of this process. Additionally, EDs who have staffing issues may have difficulty deciding between staffing an ED zone and staffing the Team Triage.

Tele-Triage[29] is another form of triage that may help overcrowded EDs. Although there are many types of Tele-Triage, it generally involves ED clinicians triaging patients through a Telehealth platform. In some models, patients will arrive in an ED triage room equipped with Telehealth technology and a remote clinician will triage the patient, perform a brief evaluation, and place orders. Other models may have ED staff in-person in the Tele-Triage who help perform vitals and other tasks. Overall, Tele-Triage can help open up another triage area to improve ED wait times to triage. Furthermore, Tele-Triage clinicians who are remote can provide triage services for multiple EDs during the same shift by using the Telehealth platform. However, Tele-Triage may take time and expenses to purchase software, train clinicians, and create a user-friendly model for patients.

Although boarding consumes staff and space, 70%–80% of ED patients are ultimately discharged. Undue emphasis is placed on the front end. Accelerating the initiation of the workup will have little effect if downstream ancillary services cannot provide timely service. Radiology turnaround time, availability and timeliness of ancillary services, and timeliness of consultants can have substantial impacts on overall turnaround time.

Vignette 1 Conclusion

The main causes of ED crowding are due to lack of hospital capacity, such as lack of discharges, more elective admissions earlier in the week, and lack of ancillary services during evenings and weekends.

Hospital-level solutions for ED overcrowding and boarding include:

- Smoothing elective admissions: You could work with the hospital teams to review elective admissions throughout the week and how they can be smoothed to decrease the large variability in elective admissions typically seen in hospitals.
- Early discharge: You could propose early discharge initiatives (i.e., discharge before noon) to help open inpatient beds before the influx of admissions from the ED that is typically seen in the afternoons.

- Weekend discharge: You could propose that the hospital increase weekend discharges by working on the barriers precluding patients from being discharged on the weekends (i.e., access to services on the weekends).
- Improving access to ancillary services: You could work with hospital-wide ancillary services that are needed for discharge, but may not be available 24/7 (i.e., ECHO, ultrasound, occupational therapy, physical therapy) to increase availability.
- Full Capacity Protocol: You could propose an FCP to place some of the patients boarding in the ED in inpatient units (hallways, conference rooms, etc.) to increase space in the ED to see new ED patients.

Vignette 2 Conclusion

Traditional ED Triage can be modified in the following ways:

- Team Triage and Tele-Triage: While working on improving the hospital capacity issues, you could implement a Team Triage and/or Tele-Triage model in your ED to improve triage delays and place orders (i.e., laboratory, radiology, medication orders) while patients are waiting to be seen in the main ED zones.

Emergency department–level solutions for ED overcrowding and boarding include:

- Focusing on turnaround time for radiology, consultants, and other ancillary services. Rapid initiation of workup accomplishes little if downstream services are not timely.

Pro-Tips

- Emergency department overcrowding and boarding are caused by lack of hospital capacity.
- Emergency department overcrowding can have significant issues, including delays in care, increased morbidity and mortality for certain illnesses, increased medical errors, and decreased satisfaction of patients and staff.
- Emergency department overcrowding can also lead to delays in triage and delays in seeing a clinician.
- The following are not long-term solutions to the ED overcrowding problem: diverting non-urgent ED patients, expanding the physical capacity of the ED, and adding ED staff.
- Potential solutions for ED overcrowding (and improving hospital capacity) are: smoothing elective admissions, early discharge, weekend discharges, and full capacity protocols.
- In overcrowded EDs, team triage and Tele-Triage can help augment the traditional nurse-only triage model.

References

1. U.S. Department of Health and Human Services – Office of the Assistant Secretary for Planning and Evaluation. Trends in the utilization of emergency department services, 2009–2018. 2021. https://aspe .hhs.gov/sites/default/files/private/pdf/2650 86/ED-report-to-Congress.pdf

2. CDC National Center for Health Statistics. Almost half of hospitals experience crowded emergency departments. September 27,

2006. www.cdc.gov/nchs/pressroom/06fac ts/hospitals.htm

3. McKenna P, Heslin SM, Viccellio P, Mallon WK, Hernandez C, Morley EJ. Emergency department and hospital crowding: causes, consequences, and cures. *Clin Exper Emerg Med.* 2019;6(3):189.

4. Singer AJ, Thode HC Jr, Viccellio P, Pines JM. The association between length of emergency department boarding and mortality. *Acad Emerg Med.* 2011;18 (12):1324–1329.

5. Weiss SJ, Ernst AA, Derlet R, King R, Bair A, Nick TG. Relationship between the National ED Overcrowding Scale and the number of patients who leave without being seen in an academic ED. *Am J Emerg Med.* 2005;23(3):288–294.

6. Reznek MA, Murray E, Youngren MN, Durham NT, Michael SS. Door-to-imaging time for acute stroke patients is adversely affected by emergency department crowding. *Stroke.* 2017;48(1):49–54.

7. Fee C, Weber EJ, Maak CA, Bacchetti P. Effect of emergency department crowding on time to antibiotics in patients admitted with community-acquired pneumonia. *Ann Emerg Med.* 2007;50(5):501–509.

8. Pines JM, Hollander JE. Emergency department crowding is associated with poor care for patients with severe pain. *Ann Emerg Med.* 2008;51(1):1–5.

9. Hwang U, Richardson L, Livote E, Harris B, Spencer N, Sean Morrison R. Emergency department crowding and decreased quality of pain care. *Acad Emerg Med.* 2008;15(12):1248–1255.

10. Horwitz LI, Green J, Bradley EH. US emergency department performance on wait time and length of visit. *YMEM.* 2010;55(2):133–141.

11. *GAO-09-347 Hospital Emergency Departments: Crowding Continues to Occur, and Some Patients Wait Longer Than Recommended Time Frames.* Washington; 2009.

12. Centers for Disease Control and Prevention. QuickStats: percentage of emergency department visits with waiting

time for a physician of > 1 hour, by race/ ethnicity and triage level – United States, 2003. *Morbidity Mortality Weekly;* 2006.

13. Pines JM, Pollack CV Jr, Diercks DB, Chang AM, Shofer FS, Hollander JE. The association between emergency department crowding and adverse cardiovascular outcomes in patients with chest pain. *Acad Emerg Med.* 2009;16 (7):617–625.

14. McCusker J, Vadeboncoeur A, Lévesque JF, Ciampi A, Belzile E. Increases in emergency department occupancy are associated with adverse 30-day outcomes. *Acad Emerg Med.* 2014; 21:1092–1100.

15. Richardson DB. Increase in patient mortality at 10 days associated with emergency department overcrowding. *Med J Aust.* 2006;184:213–216.

16. Sprivulis PC, Da Silva JA, Jacobs IG, Frazer AR, Jelinek GA. The association between hospital overcrowding and mortality among patients admitted via Western Australian emergency departments. *Med J Aust.* 2006;184:208–212.

17. Honigman LS, Wiler JL, Rooks S, Ginde AA. National study of non-urgent emergency department visits and associated resource utilization. *West J Emerg Med.* 2013;14:609–616.

18. Durand AC, Gentile S, Devictor B, Palazzolo S, Vignally P, Gerbeaux P, Sambuc R. ED patients: how nonurgent are they? Systematic review of the emergency medicine literature. *Am J Emerg Med.* 2011;29:333–345.

19. Butler C. How surgical smoothing could help ease the medical backlog created by COVID-19. CBC News. 2020, July 13. www .cbc.ca/news/canada/london/elective- surgery-wait-times-covid-surgical- smoothing-1.5641819

20. Olsen L, Saunders RS, Yong PL (eds.). *The Healthcare Imperative: Lowering Costs and Improving Outcomes: Workshop Series Summary.* National Academies Press; 2010.

21. O'Dell K. St. John's cuts errors, increases efficiency. *News-Leader,* 2006, July 5.

22. Viccellio P, Hochman KA, Semczuk P, Santora C. Right focus, right solution: how reducing variability in admission and discharge improves hospital capacity and flow. In: Litvak E (ed.). *Optimizing Patient Flow: Advanced Strategies for Managing Variability to Enhance Access, Quality, and Safety.* The Joint Commission; 2018: 97–112.

23. Garson C, Hollander JE, Rhodes KV, Shofer FS, Baxt WG, Pines JM. Emergency department patient preferences for boarding locations when hospitals are at full capacity. *Ann Emerg Med.* 2008;51:9–12.

24. Viccellio P, Zito JA, Sayage V, Chohan J, Garra G, Santora C, Singer AJ. Patients overwhelmingly prefer inpatient boarding to emergency department boarding. *J Emerg Med.* 2013;45:942–946.

25. Willard E, Carlton EF, Moffat L, Barth BE. A full-capacity protocol allows for increased emergency patient volume and hospital admissions. *J Emerg Nurs.* 2017;43:413–418.

26. Boyle A, Viccellio P, Whale C. Is "boarding" appropriate to help reduce crowding in emergency departments? *BMJ.* 2015;350:h2249.

27. Viccellio A, Santora C, Singer AJ, Thode HC Jr, Henry MC. The association between transfer of emergency department boarders to inpatient hallways and mortality: A 4-year experience. *Ann Emerg Med.* 2009;54:487–491.

28. Heslin SM, Francis A, Cloney R, Polizzo GM, Scott K, King C, Viccellio P, Rowe AL, Morley EJ. Team triage increases discharges and decreases time to discharge without increasing test ordering. *J Am Coll Emerg Phys.* 2021:2(1):e12311. doi:10.1002/emp2.12311

29. Hagland M. At Jefferson Health, a success story around ED Teletriage that offers hope. *Health Care Innovation.* 2020, March 21.

Index